The Virginia Nursing Home Survival Guide

Learn How To:

1. Select the Right Nursing Home
2. Get The Best Possible Care
3. Finance Care Without Going Broke
4. Recognize and Prevent Neglect and Abuse

By Evan H. Farr, CELA, CEA

Library of Congress Control Number: 2004195581

ISBN 0-9761821-0-6

Second Printing June 2006

Published by
Quality Legal Publications, LLC
Clifton, Virginia

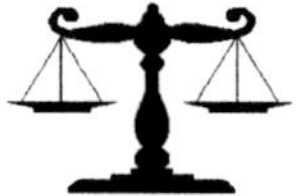

Quality Legal Publications

Printed in the United States of America by
Morris Publishing
3212 East Highway 30
P.O. Box 2110
Kearney, NE 68847
800-650-7888

Dedicated to my mother — one of the most caring persons
I have ever known — who instilled in me the
lifelong desire to help others.

Beatrice J. Farr
1933 ~ 2003

TABLE OF CONTENTS

PREFACE

Americans are living longer than ever before. At the turn of the 20th century, the average life expectancy was about 47 years. Now, in the early 21st century, life expectancy has almost doubled. According to the U.S. Census Bureau, ten thousand baby boomers (Americans born 1946 to 1964) turn 50 every day. Predictions based on the 2000 census indicate that by 2030 the number of Virginia residents aged 60 to 74 will more than double, and the number of Virginia residents aged 85 or more will increase by 150%. After age 65, Americans have a greater than 70% chance of needing some form of long term care. Tragically, Virginia currently ranks last among the 50 states in per capita health care spending for the elderly, despite the fact that Virginia is the 13th wealthiest state in the nation.

As a result of the aging of our population, we Virginians face more challenges and transitions in our lives than ever before. One of the most difficult and emotionally wrenching transitions Virginia residents must face for themselves and/or their loved ones is the move from living independently in their own homes or apartments to living in an assisted living facility or nursing home. There are many reasons why this transition is so difficult. One is the loss of home . . . often one where the person lived for many years with a lifetime of memories. Another is the loss of independence. Still another is the loss of privacy we enjoy at home, since moving to an assisted living facility or nursing home often involves sharing a room with a roommate.

The decision to move a loved one into a nursing home is one of the most difficult decisions you will ever have to make. Perhaps the reason for the move is gradual and is being made because your loved one has dementia, or a progressive disease such as Alzheimer's, and the family member can no longer care for himself or herself and requires assistance with one or more activities of daily living, such as bathing, dressing, eating, transferring from bed to chair, or using the toilet. Or perhaps the the reason for the move is sudden and is being made because your loved one has had a stroke or heart attack, or has fallen and broken a hip. Whatever the reason, most people who make the decision to move a loved one to a nursing home do so during a time of great stress.

The spouse or relative who helps a loved one transition into a nursing home faces the immediate dilemma of how to find the right nursing home. The task is no small one, and a huge sigh of relief can be heard if and when the right home is found and the loved one is moved into the nursing home. But for many, the most difficult task is just beginning: how to cope with nursing home bills that may total $5,000 to $10,000 per month or more?

The Virginia Nursing Home Survival Guide is designed to provide much-needed information and answers to the important questions you will encounter as you go through this challenging transition. These are questions that I, as an elder law attorney, deal with on a daily basis. Many of my clients have found this guide to be a valuable resource. I hope this book will be of assistance to you, too.

Evan H. Farr, CELA, CEA
Certified Elder Law Attorney, National Elder Law Foundation*
Certified Estate Advisor, National Association of Financial and Estate Planning*
Member of the National Academy of Elder Law Attorneys
Member of the AARP Legal Services Network
Owner: www.VirginiaEstatePlanning.com
Owner: www.VirginiaElderLaw.com

*Virginia has no procedure for approving certifying organizations.

chapter 1

THE CAREGIVER'S ROLE

If you're reading this book, chances are good that you are either a caregiver, or are facing the possibility of becoming a caregiver. Maybe you've been caring for your disabled spouse, or perhaps your aging parent is beginning to show signs of dementia. You're probably struggling with all kinds of difficult questions. Chances are that the person you're caring for never made any real plans for what to do in the event of physical disability or dementia.

Most family members who help their older loved ones don't see themselves as caregivers. Yet a caregiver is anyone who helps an older person with household chores, errands, personal care, or finances. Most caregivers also don't realize that caring for themselves is an important part of providing care for someone else. The simple truth is you can't be a good caregiver if you don't take care of yourself.

If you have been taking care of your spouse, perhaps you are afraid of giving up the caregiver role, even if your own health may be deteriorating as a result of the stress of having to care for your spouse. If you are an adult child, perhaps you are worried about having to provide care for a parent with diminishing health and declining capacity. It is often very difficult for an adult child to step into a relationship reversal by taking over the parental role, but that is often exactly what happens — the child must become the parent, and the parent assumes the role of the child. This transition is fraught with conflict, confusion, and pain. If you're an adult child, most likely you have a career, children, and your own family and personal limitations to deal with. How can you possibly be expected to have to take care of your parents also?

Many conflicting thoughts and emotions arise when someone is confronted with having to care for an aging parent or a disabled spouse:

- **Love and Responsibility:** a desire to provide the best care for your spouse or for your parents.
- **Fear:** fear of losing your spouse or parent; fear of losing control; fear of the unknown; fear of not being able to conserve financial assets for future needs.
- **Confusion:** not knowing what long-term care options are available, how to get the best care, how much money will need to be spent on nursing care.
- **Guilt:** for not being able to do more for your spouse or parent.
- **Anger and Frustration:** over the fact that your spouse or parent failed to plan ahead and foresee that this day might come.
- **Resentment:** over why you are the one stuck being the primary caregiver.
- **Conflict:** constant arguments with a spouse or parent who has progressive dementia.
- **Self-preservation:** worry about how much of your own limited resources must be used to provide care for your spouse or parent.

All of these feelings are normal and are neither good nor bad. Give yourself a break; being a caregiver is hard, often underappreciated work. Negative feelings do not mean you love the person any less. Allow yourself to feel how you feel and forgive yourself for any negative feelings.

CAREGIVER STRESS TEST

Which of the following are seldom true, sometimes true, often true or usually true?

- I find I can't get enough rest.
- I don't have enough time for myself.
- I don't have enough time to be with family members other than the one I care for.
- I feel guilty about my situation.
- I don't get out much anymore.
- I have conflict with the person I take care of.
- I have conflicts with other family members.
- I cry a lot.
- I worry about having enough money to make ends meet.
- I don't feel I have enough knowledge or experience to give care as well as I'd like.
- I worry about my own health.

If the response to one or more or these areas is usually true or often true, it may be time to look for help with giving care and help with taking care of yourself.

WHAT YOU CAN DO

Take charge of your life. Don't let your loved one's illness or disability always take center stage. While you might fall into a caregiving role because of an unexpected event, somewhere along the line you need to step back and consciously say "I choose to take on this caregiving role." It goes a long way toward eliminating the feeling of being a victim.

Set realistic goals. Caregiving creates many conflicting demands on your time; it is vital to set realistic goals. Recognize what you can and cannot do. Define your priorities and stick to them as much as you can. You have the right to set limits and, though it is hard, it is okay to say no.

Seek out help from family and friends. When others offer assistance, accept it and suggest specific things they can do. Some caregivers see asking for help as a sign of weakness, failure or inadequacy, when in fact it is just the opposite. Reaching out for assistance before you are beyond your limits is one characteristic of a strong person. While they might not be comfortable helping with bathing and dressing needs, friends and family can help by running errands, shopping for groceries, preparing meals or just visiting. They can call regularly, taking some pressure off you to be the primary social outlet.

Seek out appropriate geriatric medical professionals. A geriatrician is a medical doctor who is specially trained to prevent and manage the unique health concerns of older adults. Older persons may react to illness and disease differently than younger adults. Geriatricians are able to treat older patients, manage multiple disease symptoms, and develop care plans that address the special health care needs of older adults. Geriatricians are typically primary care physicians who are board-certified in either Family Practice or Internal Medicine and have also acquired the additional training necessary to obtain the Certificate of Added Qualifications in Geriatric Medicine. You can find a listing of Virginia geriatricians in **Appendix E** (page 143) of this book. You can also locate a geriatrician in your area through the Web site of either the American Medical Association (www.ama-assn.org) or the American Board of Family Medicine (www.theabfm.org).

Seek out the assistance of a Geriatric Care Manager (GCM). GCMs are professionals with degrees in one or more fields of human services (e.g., social work, psychology, nursing, or gerontology), who specialize in assisting older people and their families with long-term care arrangements. GCMs are typically independent from the resources they recommend, so they can provide an unbiased assessment of each situation. GCMs can work with families and elders prior to the need for services and can also assist in emergency situations. You can find a listing of Virginia GCMs in **Appendix F** (page 147) of this book. You can also locate a GCM in your area through the Web site of Mid-Atlantic Geriatric Care Managers Association (www.gcmonline.org).

Investigate community and professional resources such as in-home health services or adult daycare. Employ a home health aide to cook, clean and help with bathing, eating, dressing, using the bathroom and getting around the house. Check your local phonebook under "Home Health Care Providers." These are the types of services that an older parent should expect to have to pay for if they are not available for free in the community.

When you just need a short break, consider respite care. You can hire a companion to stay with your care-receiver for a few hours at a time on a regular basis to give you some time off. In addition, most nursing homes and assisted living facilities offer families the opportunity to place older relatives in their facilities for short stays. Your local area's agency on aging can help with arrangements. All Virginia Area Agencies on Aging and numerous other helpful resources are listed in **Appendix B** (page 129).

chapter 2

WHAT IS A NURSING HOME?

Nursing homes have only been around since the 1950s, but most likely you or someone close to you has spent time in a nursing home. Over the past several decades, nursing homes have become big business. The vast majority of all nursing homes are for-profit entities, and many of these are large corporations with nursing facilities in multiple states. Nursing homes generally provide three types of services:

- rehabilitation for people who are injured, sick, or disabled;
- skilled nursing and medical care;
- custodial care (help with eating, dressing, bathing, toileting, and moving about).

Like hospitals, nursing homes never close — service must be available 24 hours a day, 365 days a year with trained, licensed nursing staff always present. A nursing facility is required to maintain interdisciplinary staffing at several levels, including licensed nursing facility administrators and physician medical directors, directors of nursing services, nurses trained to provide skilled nursing care, social workers, and activities directors. They are also required to hire as staff or retain as consultants:

- A pharmacist;
- Therapists in a variety of specialties, including physical, occupational and speech therapy;
- Food service personnel, including a dietary supervisor; and

- An interdisciplinary assessment and assurance committee.

Nursing homes must be licensed under state law; more than 80% of nursing homes also choose to participate in Medicare and Medicaid, which require nursing homes to meet strict federal certification standards on quality of care, quality of life, and residents' rights. For the purposes of this book and in general consumer usage, all licensed nursing facilities are considered skilled care facilities. However, the federal government refers to non-Medicare-certified facilities as "nursing facilities" and to Medicare-certified facilities as "skilled nursing facilities" or "SNFs." The Virginia Department of Health calls facilities that do not participate in Medicaid or Medicare "non-participating facilities."

Either an entire facility or a portion of a facility can be licensed as a nursing facility. A Continuing Care Retirement Community (CCRC) offers skilled nursing facility services for its residents in a special section of the CCRC. Some hospitals may also provide skilled nursing care in a long-term care unit.

Nursing facilities use personnel at a variety of training levels, which allows patient care needs to be matched to appropriate training levels. Licensed nursing care levels in Virginia include: Licensed Practical Nurse (LPN); Registered Nurse (RN); Clinical Nurse Specialist (CNS); and Registered Nurse Practitioner (RNP).

In addition to the types of licensed and registered nurses listed above, nursing facilities may use Certified Nurse Aides, or CNAs, to provide certain basic services, although they are not licensed or registered nurses. CNAs may provide assistance with Activities of Daily Living (ADLs) such as bathing, dressing, eating, toileting, transferring, and bowel/bladder incontinence, as well as assistance with Instrumental ADLs (IADLs) which include housekeeping duties such as laundry and meal preparation. In Virginia, CNAs must: (1) complete a 120-hour training program; (2) pass a competency test within four months of being hired to work in a licensed nursing facility; and (3) be registered with the Virginia Nurse Aide Registry. To maintain its license in Virginia, a nursing facility must provide 24-hour licensed nursing care, and an RN must be on duty for at least one 8-hour shift every day of the week. Virginia licensing requirements also mandate that, at a minimum, each resident be seen by a physician at least once every 30 days for the first 90 days of care, and at least once every 60 days thereafter. Medicare-certified SNFs require a physician visit not later than 14 days after admission, and every 30 days thereafter. Additional physician visits in both nursing homes and skilled nursing facilities are according to residents' needs.

Nursing Home Goals

The goals of all nursing facilities are to: (1) rehabilitate the resident to maximum potential and enable the resident to return to independent living arrangements if possible; (2) maintain maximum rehabilitation as long as possible within the realities of age and disease; (3) delay deterioration in physical and emotional well-being; and (4) support the resident and family, physically and emotionally, when health declines to the point of death.

chapter 3
SELECTING A FACILITY

Most nursing home admissions happen under stress, often with the assistance of a hospital "discharge planner," who is typically a social worker. Discharge planners usually have general information about nursing facilities near the hospital, but they normally don't have time to learn about the actual quality of care in a given facility. If you are faced with the overwhelming task of finding the best nursing home for a loved one, where do you begin?

Although this is a job that no one wants, it can be done with forethought and confidence that the best decision was made for everyone involved. It is easier, and better for your loved one, if the first placement is to the best possible facility. Although a nursing home resident can be moved from one facility to another, this type of disruption can be very disturbing and is rarely in everyone's best interest.

To get the best possible nursing home, the first step is for the family and/or potential resident to determine what is most important to them in looking for a facility. The resident's needs and desires must be included in this evaluation. Variables such as location of the facility, whether a special care unit is available, and what types of payment sources are accepted should also be considered when beginning this process.

The next step is to identify the facilities in your area which meet the criteria you have established. The easiest place to start is in the back of this book. **Appendix A** (page 92) is a listing of all nursing homes in Virginia organized by region. If placement is not urgent, you can contact each nursing facility in your nearby area and ask for its information packet, which should include an activity calendar and a menu. You should also ask for the three most recent state annual inspection reports detailing the facility's major and minor deficiencies; nursing homes are required to make these reports available upon request. Virtually every nursing home will have some deficiencies; after all, working with extremely disabled and impaired persons is very difficult. Your local Area Agency on Aging should also have resources and helpful aids for assisting you in finding and comparing nursing homes. If you have Internet access, probably the most helpful of all resources is Medicare's Nursing Home Quality Compare Website at www.medicare.gov/NHCompare — here, you can obtain detailed inspection information about each nursing facility that interests you, comparing various government-rated "quality measures" such as: *Percent of Residents Who Have Moderate to Severe Pain, Percent of High-Risk Residents Who Have Pressure Sores, Percent of Residents Who Were Physically Restrained, and Percent of Residents Who Spend Most of Their Time in Bed or in a Chair.* The NHCompare Web site also rates the care and services that each facility provides to its residents, and allows you to view how each facility stacks up in staffing hours for each type of health care worker against the Virginia and national averages. All of the above resources, including all Virginia Area Agencies on Aging and numerous other helpful resources, are listed in **Appendix B** (page 129) and **Appendix C** (page 134).

Step three is to tour those facilities you have identified in step two. Don't schedule your visits in advance. Just show up during regular business hours. You should be able to meet with an administrative staff member, who should be able to answer all your questions. You will also want to tour a second time, in the evening or on the weekend, to see if there is a drastic difference in the atmosphere of the facility or the care being provided. It is important to tour at least two facilities so you can see the difference in the physical plant and the staff.

While you are touring the facility, pay attention to your gut feeling. Ask yourself:

- Do I feel welcome?
- How long did I have to wait to meet with someone?
- Did the admissions director ask about my family member's wants and needs?
- Is the facility clean?
- Are there any strong odors?
- Is the staff friendly?
- Do they seem to genuinely care for the residents?
- Do the staff seem to get along with each other?

Listen and observe. You can learn a lot just by watching and paying attention. And ask questions. You want to be sure that the facility is giving proactive care, not just reacting to crisis. Here are a few examples of the types of questions the staff should be able to answer:

- How do you ensure that call lights are answered promptly, regardless of your staffing?
- If my father is not able to move or turn himself, how do you ensure that he is turned and does not develop bedsores?
- How do you make sure that someone is assisted with the activities of daily living like dressing, toileting and transferring?
- Can residents bring in their own supplies?
- Can residents use any pharmacy they wish?

- How many direct care staff members do you have on each shift? Does this number exceed the minimal number that state regulations require, or do you just meet the minimum standard?
- What sources of payment do you accept?
- How long has the medical director been with your facility?
- How were your last state survey results? (Get a copy.)
- How did you correct any deficiencies and what process did you put in place to make sure you do not make these mistakes again?
- Has the state prohibited this facility from accepting new residents at any time during the last 2 years?
- What is your policy on family care planning conferences? Will you adjust your schedule to make sure that I can attend the meeting?
- Do you have a list of references I can talk with?
- Can my loved one come in for a meal to see if he/she fits in and likes the facility?

Beginning on page 14, you will find a comprehensive Nursing Home Evaluation Tool you can use when touring facilities. This tool will help you keep track of which facility you like best. You should make a separate copy of the blank form for each facility you plan to visit.

NURSING HOME EVALUATION

As you visit nursing homes, use the following form for each place you visit. Don't expect every nursing home to score well on every question. The presence or absence of any of these items does not automatically mean a facility is good or bad. Each has its own strengths and weaknesses. Simply consider what is most important to the resident and you.

Record your observations for each question by circling a number from one to five. If a question is unimportant to you or doesn't apply to your loved one, leave the evaluation area for that question blank. Then total all numbers circled for each facility.

Your ratings will help you compare nursing homes and choose the best one for your situation. The facilities with the highest scores are those on which you should focus your final attention. However, you shouldn't rely solely on the numbers. Ask to speak to family members of other residents. Also, contact the local or state ombudsman for information about the nursing home and get a copy of the facility's state inspection report from the nursing home, the agency that licenses nursing homes, or the ombudsman.

NURSING HOME EVALUATION TOOL

Name of Nursing Home: ____________________

Date Visited: ____________________

RATING SCALE				
Unacceptable	Acceptable	Average	Above Average	Excellent
1	2	3	4	5

THE BUILDING AND ITS SURROUNDINGS:

What is your first impression of the facility?	1 2 3 4 5
What is the condition of the facility's exterior paint, gutters and trim?	1 2 3 4 5
Are the grounds pleasant and well-kept?	1 2 3 4 5
Do you like the view from residents' rooms and other windows?	1 2 3 4 5
Are there appropriate areas for physical therapy and occupational therapy?	1 2 3 4 5
Do chairs and other furniture seem sturdy and difficult to tip? Are they attractive and comfortable?	1 2 3 4 5
Do patient beds in double rooms have privacy curtains?	1 2 3 4 5
Are those curtains being used by staff to protect the privacy of patients receiving treatments or assistance?	1 2 3 4 5

Is an on-site barber or beauty salon available?	1 2 3 4 5
Is an on-site library available?	1 2 3 4 5
Is an on-site computer center with high speed internet access available?	1 2 3 4 5
Is an on-site gift shop available?	1 2 3 4 5
Is an on-site general store available?	1 2 3 4 5
Do meals appear appetizing and are they served promptly at the proper times?	1 2 3 4 5
Do residents who need help eating receive adequate assistance?	1 2 3 4 5
Is the dining area clean and pleasant?	1 2 3 4 5
Is there room at and between tables for both residents and aides for those who need assistance with meals?	1 2 3 4 5
What is the level and enthusiasm of resident participation in the activities?	1 2 3 4 5
Is there a well-ventilated indoor room for smokers?	1 2 3 4 5
Is there a covered / enclosed outdoor shelter for smokers?	1 2 3 4 5
Are non-smoking rules enforced, both indoors and outdoors, in all non-smoking areas?	1 2 3 4 5
What is your impression of general cleanliness throughout the facility?	1 2 3 4 5

What is your impression of the general cleanliness and grooming of residents?	1 2 3 4 5
Does the facility smell clean?	1 2 3 4 5
Is there enough space in resident rooms and common areas for the number of residents?	1 2 3 4 5
How noisy are hallways and common areas?	1 2 3 4 5
Are common areas such as lounges and activity rooms provided?	1 2 3 4 5
Are residents allowed to bring furniture and other personal items to decorate their rooms?	1 2 3 4 5
Do residents with Alzheimer's disease live in a separate Alzheimer's unit?	1 2 3 4 5
Does the facility provide a secure outdoor area?	1 2 3 4 5
Is there a secure area where a resident with Alzheimer's can safely wander on paths?	1 2 3 4 5

THE STAFF, POLICIES AND PRACTICES:

Does the administrator know residents by name and speak to them in a pleasant, friendly way?	1 2 3 4 5
Do staff and residents communicate with cheerful, respectful attitudes?	1 2 3 4 5
Do staff and administration seem to work well with each other in a spirit of cooperation?	1 2 3 4 5

Do residents get permanent assignment of staff?	1 2 3 4 5
Do nursing assistants participate in the resident's care planning process?	1 2 3 4 5
How good is the facility's record for employee retention?	1 2 3 4 5
Does a state ombudsman visit the facility on a regular basis?	1 2 3 4 5
How likely is an increase in private pay rates?	1 2 3 4 5
Are there any additional charges not included in the daily or monthly rate?	1 2 3 4 5

QUESTIONS TO ASK THE STAFF:

Are beds available?	1 2 3 4 5
What method is used in matching roommates?	1 2 3 4 5
What is a typical day like?	1 2 3 4 5
Can residents choose what time to go to bed and wake up?	1 2 3 4 5
Are meaningful activities available that are appropriate for residents?	1 2 3 4 5
Is there an activities schedule posted? Are residents engaged in activities?	1 2 3 4 5
Can residents continue to participate in interests like gardening or contact with pets?	1 2 3 4 5

Question	Rating
Does the facility provide transportation for religious services and other activities?	1 2 3 4 5
Is a van or bus with wheelchair access available?	1 2 3 4 5
How are decisions about method and frequency of bathing made?	1 2 3 4 5
How do residents get their clothes laundered?	1 2 3 4 5
What happens when clothing or other items are missing?	1 2 3 4 5
Does the facility have a current license from the state?	1 2 3 4 5
Does the administrator have a current license from the state?	1 2 3 4 5
If Medicare and/or Medicaid coverage is needed, is the facility certified?	1 2 3 4 5
Does the facility have a formal quality assurance program?	1 2 3 4 5
Does the facility have an operating agreement with a nearby hospital for emergencies?	1 2 3 4 5
Is a physician available in an emergency?	1 2 3 4 5
Are personal physicians allowed?	1 2 3 4 5
How is regular medical attention assured?	1 2 3 4 5
How are patients and families involved in treatment plans?	1 2 3 4 5

Are specialty medical services available (e.g., dentists, podiatrists, optometrists)?	1 2 3 4 5
Does the facility report to the patient's personal physician on progress? To families?	1 2 3 4 5
What services are provided for terminally ill patients and their families?	1 2 3 4 5
Is a licensed nurse always available?	1 2 3 4 5
Does a pharmacist review patient drug regimens?	1 2 3 4 5
Are arrangement made for patients to worship or attend religious services?	1 2 3 4 5
Is physical therapy available under the direction of a licensed physical therapist?	1 2 3 4 5
Are services of an occupational therapist or speech pathologist available?	1 2 3 4 5
How are residents encouraged to participate in activities?	1 2 3 4 5
How are patient activity preferences respected?	1 2 3 4 5
Are both group and individual activities available?	1 2 3 4 5
Is a social worker available to assist residents and families?	1 2 3 4 5
Does a dietician plan menus for patients on special diets?	1 2 3 4 5

Are personal likes and dislikes taken into consideration in menu planning?	1 2 3 4 5
Are snacks available between meals?	1 2 3 4 5
Are the number of meals / snacks provided adequate?	1 2 3 4 5
Is the food preparation area separate from the dishwashing and garbage areas?	1 2 3 4 5
Is food which needs refrigeration put away promptly, and not left standing on counters?	1 2 3 4 5
Is there fresh water on bedside stands?	1 2 3 4 5
Are there hand rails in hallways and grab bars in bathrooms?	1 2 3 4 5
Are toilets convenient to bedrooms?	1 2 3 4 5
Is there a sink in each bathroom?	1 2 3 4 5
Are call bells near each toilet?	1 2 3 4 5
Are the hallways wide enough to accommodate passing wheelchairs?	1 2 3 4 5
Are the rooms large enough to allow a wheelchair to maneuver easily?	1 2 3 4 5
Is the temperature comfortable (remember many seniors prefer warmer environments)?	1 2 3 4 5
Does every patient room have a window?	1 2 3 4 5
Do all residents have closets and drawers for clothing?	1 2 3 4 5

Question	Rating
Is the atmosphere generally friendly and welcoming?	1 2 3 4 5
If residents call out for help or use a call light, do they get prompt, appropriate responses?	1 2 3 4 5
Does each resident have the same nursing assistant(s) most of the time?	1 2 3 4 5
How does a resident with problems voice a complaint?	1 2 3 4 5
How are disputes, problems, or complaints with the quality of care resolved?	1 2 3 4 5
Are residents who are able to permitted to participate in care plan meetings?	1 2 3 4 5
Does the facility have an effective resident council?	1 2 3 4 5
Is an effective family council in place?	1 2 3 4 5
Can family/staff meetings be scheduled to discuss and work out any problems that may arise?	1 2 3 4 5

Questions To Ask Yourself:

Question	Rating
Do I feel comfortable coming here/leaving my loved one here?	1 2 3 4 5
How convenient is the facility's location to me and other family members who may want to visit the resident?	1 2 3 4 5

Are there areas other than the resident's room where family members can visit?	1 2 3 4 5
Does the facility have safe, well-lighted, convenient parking?	1 2 3 4 5
Are hotels/motels nearby for out-of-town family members?	1 2 3 4 5
Are there restaurants nearby suitable for taking the resident out for a meals with family members?	1 2 3 4 5
How convenient will care planning conferences be for interested family members?	1 2 3 4 5
Is the facility convenient for the patient's personal physician?	1 2 3 4 5

Total Score: ____________

chapter 4

MOVING YOUR LOVED ONE

Once the facility has been chosen, you can take steps to make the moving process less traumatic on the resident. First, plan the admission carefully. If you know the resident becomes very difficult to deal with in the late afternoon, plan the admission for mid-morning. Next, complete the admission paperwork before your loved one actually moves into the facility. This will allow you to spend the first few hours they are there with them, getting them settled and making them feel secure in their new living environment.

Bring along some familiar items for the resident, so that his or her room will feel more like home (but keep in mind that space is limited, especially in a semi-private room). Mark every piece of clothing with a permanent laundry marker. When a facility is washing clothes for 120 people, things occasionally end up in the wrong room, but that is less likely if the item is properly marked. If you are going to do your loved one's laundry, post a sign on the closet door to notify staff, and provide a laundry bag or basket where dirty clothes can be placed.

Keep in mind that the staff of the facility is just meeting your loved one for the first time. They do not know his or her likes or dislikes, or those little nuances that make providing care go more smoothly. The best way you can help your loved one is to tell the staff, in writing, as much information as possible about your loved one, including his or her likes and dislikes, typical daily schedule, pet peeves, and so on.

Get to know the people who are caring for your loved one. Most important, stay involved. Let everyone know how much you care and how committed you are to your loved one's care. Also understand you will not help your loved one by becoming anxious or emotional. Assure him or her that although this is not an ideal situation, you will be there to make it as painless as possible.

chapter 5

How to Pay For Nursing Home Care

One of greatest concerns people have about nursing home care is how to pay for it. There are basically five ways to pay for the cost of the care provided by a nursing home:

1. **Private Pay**. This is the method many people must use at first. It means paying for the cost of a nursing home out of your own pocket. Unfortunately, with nursing home bills averaging over $5,400 per month in Northern Virginia, $4,060 throughout the rest of the Commonwealth, and topping $10,000 at some facilities, few people can afford to pay on their own for a long-term stay in a nursing home. Even those who can afford to do so often desire to explore other options — options that allow them to retain some or all of their assets for other important needs, while still permitting them to pay for nursing home care.

2. **Long Term Care Insurance.** As of the 1999 National Nursing Home Survey, private insurance accounted for only 1% of nursing home care across the country. If you have a policy with long-term care coverage, this type of coverage may go a long way toward paying the costs of the nursing home. Unfortunately, long term care insurance has only recently become popular, and most people facing a nursing home stay do not have this type of coverage in place. Many people who would like to purchase this type of coverage find that they can not afford it. How to purchase the best long-term care policy is a complicated subject that is well-worth exploring if you are in your 50s or 60s and still healthy. It

should be given serious consideration if it is affordable for you, especially in view of the new federally-mandated "Long-Term Care Partnership" which, once implemented in Virginia, should allow you to use long-term care insurance to protect an amount of assets equivalent to the premium paid for the insurance. If you are thinking about purchasing a long-term care insurance policy, an experienced elder law attorney can assist you in finding the best policy by helping you compare and contrast the numerous types of policies available and the different types and levels of coverage offered, as well as the independent ratings and financial stability of the insurance company providing the coverage. You should also discuss with an elder law attorney some of the uses of, and alternatives to, long-term care insurance, so that you have a better understanding of the cost versus benefit of such coverage.

3. **Veterans Administration**. The Veterans Administration (VA) pays for long-term care through its "Aid and Attendance" payments and through a system of federal VA nursing homes. The VA also has contracts with some community nursing homes that provide limited nursing home care. Because this payment method applies only to veterans and, even then, is extremely limited, this payment method will not be explored in this book.

4. **Medicare**. This is the national health insurance program primarily for people 65 years of age and older, those under age 65 who have been disabled for at least 24 months, and people with kidney failure. Medicare may provide some coverage for up to 100 days in a nursing facility, provided the care required is deemed "skilled nursing care," but you must meet certain strict qualification rules, which will be discussed in greater detail on page 27.

5. **Medicaid**. This is a combined federally-funded and state-funded benefit program, administered by each state, that can pay for the cost of a nursing home if certain asset and income tests are met. According to AARP, about 70 percent of nursing home residents are supported, at least in part, by Medicaid. Medicaid qualification and eligibility will be discussed in greater detail in the next chapter.

WHAT COVERAGE DOES MEDICARE PROVIDE?

Most people have a great deal of confusion between *Medicare* and *Medicaid.*

Medicare is a federally-funded and state-administered health insurance program with some limited long-term care benefits, primarily designed for individuals over age 65.

If you are enrolled in a traditional Medicare plan, and you've been in the hospital at least three days, and you are admitted directly from the hospital into a skilled nursing facility for rehabilitation or skilled nursing care, then Medicare may pay the full cost of the nursing home stay for the first 20 days, and may continue to pay part of the cost of the nursing home stay for the next 80 days — with a deductible of $119 per day[1] that you must pay privately (although there are Medicare supplement insurance policies that sometimes cover that deductible). There is also a Medicare Managed Care Plan, for which the 3-day hospital stay may not be required, and for which the deductible for days 21 through 100 is waived, provided certain strict qualifying rules are met. But whether the plan is traditional Medicare or Medicare Managed Care (MMC), the nursing home resident must be receiving daily "skilled care" and generally must continue to "improve." Medicare **will not**

---

[1] As of January 1, 2006, subject to change over time.

pay for treatment of all diseases or conditions. For example, if a long-term stay in a nursing home is due to a condition such as Alzheimer's or Parkinson's disease (which usually require custodial care, not "skilled care" and which do not "improve"), Medicare will not pay any benefits because hospitalization for these conditions is termed a "custodial nursing stay," and Medicare **does not pay** for custodial nursing home stays.

In a "best case" scenario, traditional Medicare or MMC will provide some coverage for the hospital stay and convalescence of up to 100 days for each "spell of illness" (although in our experience coverage usually falls far short of the 100-day maximum). If you recover sufficiently that you do not require a Medicare-covered care benefit for 60 consecutive days, you may be eligible for another 100 days of Medicare coverage for your next "spell of illness," but the illness or disorder must not be a chronic degenerative condition from which you will not recover.

What happens if you've used up the 100 days of coverage and still need care, or if you need a custodial nursing home stay? You're back to one of the alternatives outlined above: long-term care insurance, paying the bills with your own assets, or qualifying for Medicaid.

chapter 6

MEDICAID PLANNING

The current societal crisis posed by the increasing need for long-term care is a relatively new one. Prior to the advent of nursing homes in the 1950s, those seniors who lived into old age were typically cared for in the homes of their children. Life expectancy was such that most people died before the advent of chronic diseases such as Alzheimer's. Healthier lifestyles and advances in modern medicine have been causing Americans to live longer and longer. Unfortunately, this increased life expectancy means that Americans are often out-living their ability to care for themselves.

The governmental program that provides benefits for chronic and custodial long-term care is Medicaid. Many Americans falsely believe that Medicare will provide chronic/custodial care for themselves and their parents. These people are shocked when they learn the truth — that Medicaid, with its strict eligibility requirements, is the only governmental benefit available.

WHAT IS MEDICAID?

Medicaid is a benefits program that is funded by the federal and state governments and administered by each state. While the rules for eligibility vary from state to state, the primary benefit of Medicaid is that it will pay for long-term care in a nursing home once you have qualified. As mentioned previously, according to AARP about 70 percent of nursing home residents are supported, at least in part, by Medicaid.

In our lifetime, Medicaid has effectively become the long-term care insurance of the middle class because most people cannot afford to pay the Virginia average of $4,060 per month ($5,403 in Northern

Virginia) indefinitely for nursing home care. As the primary source of nursing home funding in the United States, Medicaid, created in 1965 under President Lyndon Johnson, is, according to Senator Jay Rockefeller IV, one of the Federal Government's three "social contracts" with America — the other two being Social Security (which provides retirement income for older Americans), and Medicare (which provides health coverage). In 2005 Senator Rockefeller, then the ranking member of the Senate Finance Committee's Subcommittee on Health Care, in marking the 40th anniversary of the Medicaid program, stated that

> "President Johnson's noble concept was not just a Democratic ideal; it had been an inspiration shared throughout the early part of the century by legislators and presidents from both parties. And since the signing of the landmark legislation, administrations - both Republican and Democratic - have fought to preserve the Medicaid mission of providing healthcare for the nation's most vulnerable citizens.
>
> "Sadly, in the past few years, we have seen a misguided, darker view of Medicaid emerge - one that loses sight of its original goal and underlying moral framework. Medicaid has become a scapegoat for the larger ills facing our entire healthcare system. But Medicaid isn't the problem. . . . Taking care of our most vulnerable people is a moral obligation.
>
> "Our representative democracy has a responsibility to do for the future what we have repeatedly done in the past: protect, preserve, and strengthen Medicaid."

How To Apply For Virginia Medicaid

Applications for Virginia Medicaid are filed with the appropriate local office of the Department of Social Services or Department of Family Services (hereinafter referred to as the "Department") in the city or county where the applicant lives; assuming the applicant is already living in a nursing home, then the application is submitted to the Department in the city or county where the nursing home is located, regardless of where the applicant lived prior to entering the nursing home and regardless of whether the applicant lived in Virginia prior to entering the nursing home. A list of all local Departments in Virginia can be found online at www.dss.state.va.us/localagency. A Medicaid application must be filled out and signed by the applicant, the applicant's attorney, the applicant's agent under a durable power of attorney, or the applicant's legal guardian, conservator, or other authorized representative. A face-to-face interview is not required. Among other things, applicants for Medicaid are asked to:

- Provide Social Security numbers.
- Confirm Virginia residency.
- Confirm U.S. citizenship or provide documentation of alien status.
- Disclose and verify all income and assets.
- Disclose and verify all transfers of assets during the 60-month period prior to application.
- Submit income tax returns for the past 3 years.
- Submit all bills for medical services and nursing home care received in the past three months.

Once a completed application is received, it will be a assigned to an eligibility worker at the local Department, who will typically make an initial review of the application and supporting documentation and send the applicant a checklist of additional required information and documentation. If the eligibility worker has questions that can not be easily answered by written documentation, a face-to-face meeting may be requested. Unfortunately, however, the local Department is often extremely busy and/or short-handed, and applications will frequently be denied without the applicant having been given the opportunity to submit the missing information or verifications.

For each Medicaid application, the local Department is required to issue a written determination as to whether the applicant is deemed eligible for Virginia's Medicaid Program within 45 days (90 days if a disability determination is needed) from the date the application was filed. If the applicant disagrees with the decision made by the local Department, an appeal may be filed within thirty days.

WHY SEEK LEGAL ADVICE FOR MEDICAID?

Meeting the eligibility rules for Medicaid benefits requires passing certain very strict tests regarding income and assets. In addition to being strict, the Medicaid eligibility rules are extremely complicated and confusing. The United States Supreme Court has called the Medicaid laws "an aggravated assault on the English language, resistant to attempts to understand it." *Schweiker v. Gray Panthers*, 453 U.S. 34, 43 (1981). The United States Court of Appeals for our own Fourth Circuit (just below the U.S. Supreme Court), in a case arising out of Virginia, has called the Medicaid Act one of the "most completely impenetrable texts within human experience" and "dense reading of the most tortuous kind." *Rehab. Association of Virginia v. Kozlowski*, 42 F.3d 1444, 1450 (4th Cir. 1994).

Due to tremendous complexity of the Medicaid laws, the Medicaid application process is also extremely complicated, and many persons who file for Medicaid without professional assistance will wind up with the application being rejected for a variety of reasons. Rejection often occurs due to financial issues — either excess resources, excess income, or improperly-timed gifts or transfers. Rejection in many cases is due to missing or incomplete information or verifications. Applications are also sometimes improperly rejected by an eligibility worker (most of whom are underpaid and overworked) who has not had the time to carefully and thoroughly review the application and verifications, or who has improperly applied the legal or financial requirements for eligibility.

Worse yet, an application that is filed at the wrong time can result not only in rejection, but in the imposition of significant penalties against the applicant that could have been avoided by a more timely filing. For these and many other reasons, an experienced elder law attorney should always be hired to represent the applicant through the entire Medicaid process — including planning for eligibility, preparing and filing the application, working with the local Department during the application and verification process, filing an appeal when necessary, and representing the applicant in connection with any required hearings and appeals.

Without proper planning and legal advice from an experienced elder law attorney, many people spend much more than they should on long-term care, and unnecessarily jeopardize their future care and well-being, as well as the security of their family.

What Type Of Planning Can Be Done?

The type of planning done by most experienced elder law attorneys is known by many names — it may be called *Asset Protection*, *Long-term Care Planning*, *Life Care Planning*, or *Medicaid*

Planning. What is the goal of this type of planning? The goals differ from person to person and family to family. Generally, for a married couple the most important goal is to ensure that the spouse remaining at home is able to live the remaining years of his or her life in utmost dignity, without having to suffer a drastic reduction in his or her standard of living. For a single or widowed client, the most important goal is typically to be able to enjoy the highest quality of life possible in the event of an extended nursing home stay. When there is an adult child or grandchild who is disabled, the primary goal is typically to protect assets to be used for the benefit of that disabled family member who is often also receiving Medicaid and Social Security Disability benefits. Money that is protected through proper planning can be used to provide a nursing home resident with an enhanced level of care and a better quality of life while in a nursing home and receiving Medicaid benefits. For instance, protected assets can be used to hire a private nurse or a private health aide — someone to provide one-on-one care to the resident — to help the resident get dressed, to help the resident get to the bathroom, to help the resident at mealtime, and to act as the resident's eyes, ears and advocate.

Money that is sheltered through proper planning can also be used to purchase things for the nursing home resident or disabled child that are not covered by Medicaid — such as special medical devices, upgraded wheel chairs, transportation services, trips to the beauty salon, etc.

Lastly, some parents do have a strong desire to leave a financial legacy for their children, particularly if there is a disabled child or someone who needs special financial help.

Exempt Assets and Countable Assets: What Must Be Spent?

To qualify for Medicaid, applicants must pass some very strict tests on the type and amount of assets they can keep. To understand how Medicaid works, one first needs to learn to differentiate what are known as "exempt assets" from "countable" assets.

Exempt assets are those that Medicaid does not take into account. In Virginia, that currently includes:

- The applicant's principal residence (however, after the nursing home resident has been in the nursing home for six months of continuous institutionalization, the resident's home will become a countable resource unless the resident's spouse or other dependent relatives live in the home);
- Personal possessions, such as clothing, furniture, and jewelry;
- One motor vehicle, without regard to value;
- Property used in a trade or business;
- Certain prepaid burial arrangements;
- Term life insurance policies;
- A life estate in real estate (however, the transfer rules on life estates are very complicated and must be carefully observed);
- IRS Code d(4)(A) and d(4)(C) Special Needs Trusts; and

- Any assets that are considered inaccessible for one reason or another.

All other assets are generally "countable" assets, technically called "resources." Basically all money and property, and any item that can be valued and turned into cash, is a countable asset unless it is listed above as exempt. This includes:

- Cash, savings and checking accounts, credit union share and draft accounts;
- Certificates of deposit;
- U.S. Savings Bonds;
- Individual Retirement Accounts (IRAs), Keogh plans, 401(k) and 403(b) accounts;
- Nursing home accounts;
- Prepaid funeral contracts that can be canceled;
- Certain trusts (depending on the terms of the trust);
- Real estate other than the primary residence;
- Any additional motor vehicles;
- Boats or recreational vehicles;
- Stocks, bonds, or mutual funds; and
- Land contracts or mortgages held on real estate;

An unmarried applicant may have no more than $2,000 in "countable" assets in his or her name in order to be "resource eligible" for Medicaid.

Does this mean that if you need Medicaid assistance, you'll have to spend nearly all of your assets to qualify? No — there are numerous different strategies that can be employed to legally and ethically protect assets. An experienced elder law attorney can walk a family through the different strategies that apply to a particular situation and discuss these strategies with the family to determine which ones are appealing and viable under the circumstances, and which strategies are inappropriate. Consider the following case study:

CASE STUDY: MEDICAID PLANNING FOR A SINGLE PERSON

Jill is worn out. Three years ago her mother died, and for the past two years she's been caring for her aging father, Harry. At first it was little things . . . grocery shopping, trips to the doctor, and help with medications. But as Harry's health has deteriorated, Jill's burden has increased. The last six months have been brutal because Jill finally had to move Harry to a nursing home — Harry couldn't safely stay at home by himself any more.

Jill thought her job would be easier once the nursing home staff took over, but it hasn't turned out that way. She's the oldest daughter, so she still feels responsible, even though the nursing home is now responsible for Harry's day-to-day care. Between visiting Harry every day, paying Harry's bills, and handling other matters involving her dad, Jill spends at least two hours a day on her dad's affairs.

Jill is running herself ragged, and Harry is running out of money. There's only about $90,000 left, and at $6,000 per month for the nursing home, Jill knows the money will only last about another 15 months. Once the money runs out, how can Jill pay for Harry's care? Jill has heard that Medicaid will cover the nursing home, but she's also heard that Medicaid won't cover everything. "What then?" she asks, distraught. "Is there anything else I can do?"

Yes, there are steps she can take. Given her high degree of involvement, a *personal care contract*, sometimes called a *life care agreement*, should be considered. Jill and Harry can enter into a formal agreement in which Jill becomes Harry's care manager. Even though Harry is in a nursing home, if the agreement is properly drawn, Harry can pay Jill for her care management services.

For example, if Jill spends about 2 hours a day caring for Harry, that's about 60 hours per month (30 days per month times 2 hours per day). If the personal care agreement specifies that Jill's time can be compensated at the rate of $15 per hour, that's $900 per month for Jill's services. In and of itself, that doesn't sound exciting. However, if Jill and Harry enter into a properly drawn life care agreement, Harry can agree to have Jill act as his care manager for as long as Harry lives. In other words, Harry can pay Jill $10,800 per year ($900 per month times 12 months), and Harry can make this payment in a lump sum for Harry's life expectancy. So, if Harry has a life expectancy of 8 years, he can pay Jill $86,400 ($10,800 per year times 8 years) up front, in one lump sum. This arrangement will permit Jill to provide her father with the care he needs, and still allows Harry to qualify for Medicaid, which solves Jill's and Harry's dilemma.

Please note that the scenario outlined above is the "short version." This sort of planning must be handled in a very specific manner, and it's important to seek the assistance of a knowledgeable elder law attorney before attempting to use this method, or any of the other planning methods that are available.

MEDICAID PLANNING FOR MARRIED COUPLES

Federal law provides some basic built-in protection for married couples. The Medicare Catastrophic Coverage Act of 1988 contained "spousal impoverishment" provisions that offer assistance to married couples. The law's intent was to change the eligibility requirements for Medicaid where one spouse needs nursing home care but the other spouse remains at home in the community. This law recognizes that it makes little sense to impoverish both spouses when only one needs to qualify for Medicaid assistance for nursing home care.

***Division of Countable Assets and "Spend Down*.**" To begin the division of assets, the couple must list all of their countable assets (exempt assets, as discussed above, are not included). The countable assets are then divided, for purpose of calculation, into equal halves. One-half of said countable assets, up to $99,540[2], is then allocated to the at-home spouse (technically called the "community spouse," though we will use the term "at-home spouse" throughout this book for clarity). This amount that is allocated to the "community spouse" is called the "Community Spouse Resource Allowance" or CSRA. The other half of the countable assets is allocated to the nursing home spouse, and must be "spent down" until only $2,000 remains, at which time the nursing home spouse will then qualify for Medicaid. As a practical matter, when married couples in Virginia do proper planning, all assets should almost always be transferred to the at-home spouse prior to the spouse in need entering the nursing home. For example, if a couple owns $100,000 in countable assets just prior to the date the applicant enters the nursing home, all of these assets would generally be transferred to the at-home spouse. The applicant will be eligible for Medicaid once the couple's combined

---

[2] All dollar amounts on this and the next page are effective as of January 1, 2006, and are subject to change over time.

assets (now all in name of the at-home spouse) have been reduced to a combined figure of $52,000 ($2,000 for the applicant plus $50,000 for the at-home spouse). If the couple owned $200,000 in combined assets, the spouse entering the nursing home would not become eligible for Medicaid until their combined assets were reduced to $101,540 ($2,000 for the applicant plus a maximum of $99,540 for the at-home spouse). There is also a minimum resource allowance for the community spouse in the amount of $19,908.

The determination of the amount of the couple's assets is made as of the first day of the month that the applicant enters the nursing home. This is often called the "snapshot date." It may be advantageous for the couple to have as much money as possible in their names on the snapshot date, up to $201,080 ($99,540 x 2 + $2,000) so that the amount the at-home spouse is allowed to keep will be as high as possible.

After the spouse in the nursing home qualifies for Medicaid long-term care assistance, the assets of the at-home spouse are no longer deemed available to the institutionalized spouse.

Calculation of Minimum Monthly Income. Each state also establishes a monthly income floor for the at-home spouse, called the Minimum Monthly Maintenance Needs Allowance, or MMMNA. In Virginia, the MMMNA ranges from a low of $1,603.75 per month to a high of $2,377.50 per month, and cannot exceed $2,488.50 unless a court orders support in a greater amount. In Virginia, the MMMNA is calculated as follows:

(1) $1,603.75 plus

(2) The Excess Shelter Allowance, which equals the amount by which rent, mortgage payments, taxes, insurance, and utilities exceed the "Excess Shelter Standard" of $481.13. There is a standard utility allowance in the amount of $227 for a household of 1 to 3 members, and $282 for a household of 4 or more 3 members.

If the at-home spouse's income falls below his or her MMMNA, the shortfall can be made up from the nursing home spouse's income. That is, the at-home spouse may take as much income of the nursing home spouse as is necessary to reach the MMMNA, which should avoid the necessity of the at-home spouse dipping into savings each month, which might result in gradual impoverishment.

For example, assume (1) that the at-home spouse's sole source of income is $800 per month in Social Security benefits and (2) that her MMMNA has been calculated to be the Virginia minimum of $1,603.75 . Since she is entitled to a minimum monthly income of $1,603.75, but only receives $800, she is entitled to collect the difference of $803.75 every month from the nursing home spouse's Social Security check. The rest of the nursing home spouse's income will be paid to the nursing home, to partially cover the cost of her husband's care.

$1,603.75	At-home spouse's maximum income allowance, as determined by formula
($800.00)	Less the at-home spouse's actual income, from Social Security
$803.75	The shortfall, which will be paid to her from her spouse's Social Security.

On the other hand, if the at-home spouse's gross monthly income is $2,000, he or she is expected to contribute $15 per month to the cost of the nursing-home spouse's care. This monthly payment by the at-home spouse increases by $10 per month for each additional $100 of monthly income. For example, if the at-home spouse's gross monthly income is $2,300, he or she will be expected to contribute $45 per month ($10 times 3 = $30 + $15 = $45). Note that if the at-home spouse is entitled to receive an allowance from the nursing home spouse, the at-home spouse does not have an expected contribution.

There are many other planning alternatives that a married couple can pursue. Though some families do spend virtually all of their savings on nursing home care, Medicaid laws do not require it. There are numerous legal and ethical strategies which can be used, with the assistance of a knowledgeable elder law attorney, to protect family financial security. These strategies include: prepayment of real estate taxes; payment of certain types of debts at the proper time; conversion of countable assets to non-countable assets; payment for home improvements; purchase of a new home; transfer of the residence to the at-home spouse; transfer of the residence to a disabled child; transfer of financial assets to the at-home spouse; purchase of pre-paid funeral arrangements; purchase of a new car; creation of a life care agreement; creation of a life estate in real estate; creation of an irrevocable trust; purchase of a special type of commercial annuity; or by obtaining a reverse mortgage. Consider the following case studies.

Case Study: Advanced Medicaid Planning For Married Couples

Ralph and Betty, both age 82, were high school sweethearts who lived in Annandale, Virginia their entire adult lives. They purchased their modest-sized home for $22,000 and now the land alone is worth over $450,000. Two weeks ago, their son and daughter threw Ralph and Betty a surprise 60th anniversary party. Yesterday, Ralph, who has Alzheimer's, wandered away from home. The police found him, hours later, sitting on a curb, talking incoherently, with a broken hip. They took him to Inova Fairfax Hospital. Now the family doctor has told Betty that she needs to place Ralph in a nursing home. The nursing home closest to their house charges $220 per day — approximately $6,600 per month. Ralph and Betty grew up during the Depression, and always tried to save something each month. Their financial assets, totaling $140,000 (not including the real estate), are as follows:

Savings	$65,000.00
CDs	$35,000.00
Money Market	$27,000.00
Checking	$13,000.00
Total	$140,000.00

Ralph gets a Social Security check for approximately $1,000 each month; Betty's check is $450. Her eyes fill with tears as she says, "Ralph's dad lived to age 95, and spent his last 7 years in a nursing home. If we have to pay $6,600 to the nursing home every month, our entire life savings will be gone in a little over two years! And then I'll have to sell the home and will have nowhere to live." Betty's also afraid she won't be able to pay her monthly bills because a friend told her that the nursing home will be entitled to all of Ralph's Social Security check.

There is good news for Ralph and Betty. It's possible they Betty can get to keep everything — all of their assets and all of the income — and still arrange for the Virginia Medicaid program to pay for Ralph's nursing home costs.

To apply for Medicaid, Betty will have to go through her local Department of Social Services — DSS (or, in some jurisdictions, the Department of Family Services — DFS). If she does things strictly according to the way DSS tells her, Ralph will qualify for Medicaid once their joint assets have been reduced to $72,000 ($70,000 which she is allowed to keep as her CSRA — since their total assets are $140,000 — and $2,000 which Ralph is allowed to keep), and she will be entitled to a Minimum Monthly Maintenance Needs Allowance to pay her own monthly expenses. As we have already seen, the Minimum Monthly Maintenance Needs Allowance starts at a low of $1,603.75 per month, so Betty would be entitled to all of Ralph's income. But the situation can actually be much better than this. Ralph and Betty can also transfer Ralph's half of the joint family assets to Betty, so that all $140,000 of the family assets are in Betty's name. This must be done quickly, while Ralph is still having some "good days," unless Ralph previously has given a power of attorney to make this transfer. Then, instead of having to spend down Ralph's $68,000, Betty can use Ralph's $68,000 to purchase a special type of irrevocable commercial annuity — sometimes called a Medicaid Annuity — that pays income to Betty only — and will not be a countable resource in determining Medicaid eligibility for Ralph. This annuity can be set up to pay income to Betty for at little as 1 or 2 years, or for as long as Betty's life expectancy. Since Betty desperately needs additional income, her annuity will be set up to pay her income each month for the remainder of her life expectancy.

What about their marital home? If it stays titled jointly, Betty could predecease Ralph and the home would then pass to Ralph, at which time the house would have to be sold and the proceeds used to pay the nursing home until Ralph has spent all of those proceeds and can then reapply for Medicaid once his total assets have been depleted back down to $2,000. To prevent this possibility, the home can and should be deeded to Betty, so if Betty were to die before Ralph, the house will pass to the children. The children can then sell the house and hold the proceeds from the sale for the use and benefit of their father, to supplement Ralph's care in the nursing home while still allowing Ralph to remain on Medicaid.

Case Study: Advanced Medicaid Planning For A Single or Widowed Individual

Five years later, after Ralph's death, Betty is becoming concerned that she may one day wind up in a nursing home like Ralph. She has her Social Security income, and Ralph's survivor benefit, and the income from the Medicaid Annuity, but her income is still not nearly enough to afford the monthly cost of nursing care. She's afraid that her home will have to be sold and all of the proceeds spent to pay for her nursing home care. Although this is what DSS will tell her, there are numerous other options. With proper planning, Betty can protect some or all of the value of her home while still continuing to live in the home as long as she is able to. One method of accomplishing this goal would be to transfer the remainder interest in her home to her children while keeping a life estate, and either keeping enough financial assets to pay for a nursing home stay during the period of ineligibility caused by the transfer of the remainder interest, or entering into a life care agreement. There are several other methods as well, and an experienced elder law attorney can walk the family through the different options and select which options make the most sense under the circumstances.

chapter 7

Frequently Asked Questions About Medicaid

Question: Is it *legal* to transfer or retitle assets in an attempt to qualify for Medicaid?

Answer: Yes, it is absolutely legal. There are no laws prohibiting the transfer or re-titling of assets. However, transfers must be made very carefully, because a Medicaid applicant who has made uncompensated transfers within 5 years (or 3 years if the transfer was made prior to Feb. 8, 2006) of applying for Medicaid will face a "period of ineligibility" for Medicaid based on the amount of the transfer divided by the average cost of a month of nursing home care in the applicant's geographic area. For example, in Northern Virginia (the counties of Arlington, Fairfax, Loudoun and Prince William, and the cities of Alexandria, Fairfax, Falls Church, Manassas and Manassas Park), every $5,403 given away during the 5 years prior to a Medicaid application creates a one month "period of ineligibility" (in the rest of Virginia, every $4,060 gift creates the same waiting period), which period of ineligibility may be longer than 5 years. For example, if an applicant in Fairfax County gives her house, worth $500,000, to her children two years prior to her nursing home admission, the applicant would be ineligible for Medicaid for at least 92 months ($500,000 ÷ $5,403 = 92.5).

Question: Is it *ethical* to transfer and retitle assets in an attempt to qualify for Medicaid?

Answer: Yes, it is absolutely ethical and moral; in fact, it is the "right" thing to do if a family is concerned about the long-term care of a loved one. From a moral and ethical standpoint, Medicaid planning is no different from income tax planning and estate planning.

Income tax planning involves trying to find all of the proper and legal deductions, credits, and other tax savings that you are entitled to — taking maximum advantage of existing laws. Income tax planning also involves investing in tax-free bonds, retirement plans, or other tax-favored investment vehicles, all in an effort to minimize what you pay in income taxes and maximize the amount of money that remains in your control to be used to benefit you and your family.

Estate planning involves trying to plan your estate to minimize the amount of estate taxes and probate taxes that your estate will have to pay to the government, again taking maximum advantage of the existing laws. Similar to income-tax planning, estate planning is a way to minimize what your estate pays in taxes and maximize the amount of money that remains in your estate to be used to benefit your family.

Similarly, Medicaid planning involves trying to find the best methods to transfer, shelter, and protect your assets in ways that take maximum advantage of existing laws, all in an effort to minimize what you pay and maximize the amount of money that remains in your control to be used to benefit you and your family.

Like income-tax planning and estate planning, Medicaid planning requires a great deal of extremely complex knowledge due in part to constantly-changing laws, so you need to work with an experienced elder law attorney who knows the rules and can advise you properly.

Question: If someone transfers assets, when does the Medicaid "period of ineligibility" start — when the transfer is made or when the applicant applies for Medicaid?

Answer: The answer to this question depends on when the transfer was made. For a transfer made prior to February 8, 2006, the old law will apply and the period of ineligibility will begin when the transfer was made. For a transfer made after February 8, 2006, the new law will presumably apply and the period of ineligibility will begin when the applicant applied for Medicaid, assuming the applicant is otherwise eligible for Medicaid *but for* the application of the period of ineligibility.

Question: How much of my assets can be protected?

Answer: This varies from client to client and depends on the situation and the specific goals and desires of the client and the client's family. In general, an experienced elder law attorney should be able to protect anywhere from forty percent (40%) to one-hundred percent (100%) of a person's assets, depending on the situation. As a general rule, the earlier someone begins the planning process, the more assets that person will be able to protect.

Question: I've heard you can't do Medicaid planning within three years of entering a nursing home — is this true? And does the new law mean you have to do this type of planning five years prior to entering a nursing home?

Answer: No and No. This was a myth under the old law and remains a myth under the new law. As we have already stated, the law imposes a calculated period of ineligibility for certain types of transfers made prior to applying for Medicaid; however, an experienced elder law attorney will be mindful of these laws and will be careful to comply fully with and work within the law, sometime even making transfers intentionally to create a period of ineligibility. Plus, there are several different planning strategies that can be implemented at any time — even after someone has already entered a nursing home — and will not trigger any period of ineligibility. Because of the complexities of this type of planning, many of the strategies used and transfers made as part of a Medicaid plan are often very time sensitive, and you must always be sure to follow your attorney's instructions carefully.

Question: If I added a child's name to my bank account (or the title to my home) more than 5 years ago, is it now protected from having to be spent for the nursing home?

Answer: No. The entire amount in a joint bank account is still counted as belonging to you unless you can prove some or all of the money was actually contributed by the child whose name is on the account. This rule applies to all assets, including real estate. Moreover, joint ownership with children can be disastrous for a number of reasons unrelated to Medicaid transfer rules. For example, your accounts, once in joint ownership with a child, will be vulnerable to the debts and liabilities of that child. Thus, if your child is in an automobile accident, your property could be at risk; or if your child has a business setback, runs up large debts, or goes through a bankruptcy or divorce, your home will be at risk. Also, because jointly-owned assets will pass directly to the co-owner when you die, and not through your Will or Trust, titling assets in joint ownership may unintentionally disinherit your other children.

Question: Can't I just give all of my assets away?

Answer: The answer is "maybe" — but only if you do it the right way and at the right time. If assets are given away at the wrong time and/or in the wrong amount, the law provides for a penalty — a period of ineligibility for Medicaid — based on the amount of the transfer.

Question: Doesn't federal law allow me to give away $10,000 per year to my children?

Answer: Yes. In fact, the limit has gone up to $12,000 — the Federal Gift Tax laws allow you to give away up to $12,000 per year to anyone you want. You and your spouse may each give an unlimited number of these $12,000 gifts per year. So, for example, if you have 4 children and 8 grandchildren, you could give away up to \$144,000 each year (\$12,000 x 12) if you each gave \$12,000 to each child and grandchild. However, even though the Federal Gift Tax laws allow you to give away up to \$12,000 per year to as many people as you wish *without gift tax consequences*, Medicaid laws still apply to these gifts, meaning that these gifts will result in a penalty — a period of ineligibility for Medicaid in Northern Virginia of more than two months per \$12,000 gift (\$12,000 ÷ \$5,403 = 2.22). So, your \$144,000 annual gift would actually result in more than two years of ineligibility for Medicaid.

Question: Does giving money to my church or other charities create a penalty?

Answer: Yes. Giving away money to charity is treated the same as giving away money to your children or grandchildren. There is no exception for gifts made to charity. Many people who apply for Medicaid are horrified to discover that they are penalized for having been good citizens and having given money to charities.

Question: If I gave assets away and created a period of ineligibility for Medicaid, can the person to whom I gave the assets return the assets to me and eliminate the period of ineligibility?

Answer: Yes — the general rule is that a transfer can be cured by the return of the transferred asset. In fact, there is a potential planning strategy under the new law that is based on the partial return of transferred assets. However, because the regulations giving effect to the new law have yet to be written, it is not clear whether this new strategy will work.

Question: Are there any assets that can be transferred without resulting in a period of ineligibility?

Answer: Yes. There are transfers to certain recipients that will not trigger a period of Medicaid ineligibility. These exempt recipients include:

(1) A spouse (or anyone else for the spouse's benefit);

(2) A blind or disabled child;

(3) A trust for the benefit of a blind or disabled child; or

(4) A trust for the benefit of a disabled individual under age 65 (even for the benefit of the applicant under certain circumstances).

Question: Are there any special rules that apply to the transfer of a family home?

Answer: Yes. There are special exceptions that apply with regard to the transfer of a family home. In addition to being able to make the transfers without penalty to one's spouse or blind or disabled child, or into trust for other disabled beneficiaries, the applicant may freely transfer his or her home to:

(1) A child under age 21 (though transferring to a child under 18 can be very dangerous);

(2) A sibling who has lived in the home during the year preceding the applicant's institutionalization and who already holds an equity interest in the home; or

(3) A "caretaker child," defined as a child of the applicant who lived in the house for at least two years prior to the applicant's entry into a nursing home and who during that period provided such care that the applicant did not need to move to a nursing home. Very strict proof requirements are needed to obtain this exception.

Question: Can I really be forced to sell my home in order to qualify for Medicaid?

Answer: Yes — without proper advance planning, many Medicaid applicants find themselves forced to sell their homes in order to qualify for Medicaid.

Under Virginia Medicaid, as previously explained, the home is an exempt asset only if there is an at-home spouse living in the home.

Otherwise, the home must be sold six months after qualifying for Medicaid, and the sales proceeds must then be used to pay for the nursing home.

Fortunately, there are many ways in Virginia to protect the equity in a home, but since the Medicaid rules are complex and constantly changing, you will need to seek help from an experienced elder law attorney to help you in your planning.

Question: You mentioned earlier that a life estate in real estate is an exempt asset — what is a life estate and how can it be used in Medicaid Planning?

Answer: Life estate deeds are used in Virginia for many different purposes, including Medicaid planning and avoiding probate. A life estate in real estate is a type of "split interest" ownership based on time, similar in concept to a timeshare. If you own a timeshare, you have the exclusive right to use your timeshare property during your period of ownership, typically a certain week each year. When you own a life estate, you have the right to live in the property for the rest of your life, and your ownership interest terminates upon your death. For example, a mother can transfer a home to her daughter by deeding to the daughter what is called a "remainder interest" in the property, with the mother keeping a "retained life estate," which will allow the mother the right to live in the home for her remaining lifetime and to be considered the owner of the home for most purposes. In this situation, the deed would normally be written so that the mother will still be responsible for the payment of all taxes, insurance and maintenance on the home.

One common Medicaid planning strategy under the old Medicaid law was the purchase of a life estate in the home of a child, even if the parent never lived in the home. Although the new Medicaid law considers purchase of a life estate to be a penalized transfer if the applicant does not reside in the home for at least a year, the new law appears to allow a parent to purchase a child's home and then sell the child a remainder interest in the home, thereby accomplishing the same goal. However, because the regulations giving effect to the new law have not yet been written, it is not clear whether this new strategy will work.

Another common Medicaid planning strategy involves the gift of a remainder interest. A gift of a remainder interest in real estate has many advantages over an outright gift of real estate by a regular deed: 1) the parent, as the owner of the life estate, will continue to qualify for any property tax exemptions such as veterans and senior citizens exemptions that were available prior to the transfer; 2) the parent will not lose the legal right to live in the property, sell the property, or rent the property; 3) the children can't make the parent move out; 4) the children's creditors or bankruptcy trustee can't take possession of the property; 5) capital gains when the children sell the home will be calculated on a stepped-up basis, which is the value at the date of the parent's death rather than the parent's original cost basis; and 6) since the value of the remainder interest is lower than the full value of the house, a gift of a remainder interest will result in a shorter Medicaid penalty period than a transfer of the entire house.

To determine exactly how a gift of a remainder interest will affect eligibility for Medicaid, the look-back period and the value of the transfer must be considered. The transfer is not considered to be for the full value of the house but only the "remainder interest" in the house. The remainder interest is the right that the children have to receive the home automatically upon the death of the parent. The value of the remainder interest is calculated using special actuarial tables that determine the parent's life expectancy. The number of months of ineligibility is calculated by dividing the value of the transfer by the average monthly cost of nursing home care — $5,403 per month in Northern Virginia, $4,060 throughout the rest of the Commonwealth.

The Department cannot require an applicant to liquidate the life estate or to rent the life estate interest property. However, if the property is rented, the net rental income must go to the nursing home resident and will be counted in determining eligibility for Medicaid.

If the property is sold during the lifetime of the parent, how the sales proceeds are treated depends on how the deed is worded. The deed can be worded so that the parent will continue to have a life estate in any replacement real estate and/or in the proceeds of sale. If the parent receives income from the invested proceeds, that income will be counted in determining eligibility for Medicaid. Or, the deed can be worded so that the life estate is terminated upon sale of the property, in which case the parent's portion of the proceeds will be a countable resource for determining Medicaid eligibility.

chapter 8

HOW TO GET THE BEST POSSIBLE CARE

Once you find a nursing home placement for your loved one, you can begin the process of easing the transition from one level of care to another. If you have been providing some or all of your loved one's care, you will notice a change in your role. Rather than functioning as a caregiver, you will become a care advocate. You will still be caring for your loved one, but in a new way.

Your key roles will be to participate in planning your loved one's care, communicating frequently with the facility staff, and ensuring that your loved one gets the best possible care in the new environment. If your loved one has assets set aside that have been properly protected using some of the techniques discussed in the previous chapter, these assets can now be used to enhance the level and quality of care that will be provided to your loved one. You can use these protected assets to hire a private caregiver or a Geriatric Care Manager, to purchase the best medical equipment, and to hire the best doctors for your loved one.

CARE PLANNING

Federal law requires every long-term care facility to create a care plan. The care plan begins with a baseline assessment, which should occur within two weeks after a resident moves into the new facility, by a team from the nursing home (which may include a doctor, nurse, social worker, dietician, and physical, occupational, or recreational therapist). This team will use information provided by the resident and the family about the resident's medical and emotional needs to generate this baseline assessment, which then becomes the yardstick against which the caregivers can measure the resident's progress.

You can help by making a list of your loved one's medical, psychological, spiritual, and social needs, as well as his or her preferences and usual routine. For example, you might give the staff the following type of information: "Dad likes to listen to classical music on the radio as he falls asleep" or "Mom's always been a night-owl; she goes to sleep at around 1 a.m. and wakes up at 10am." You should also note signs of depression, or symptoms of dementia. Since the assessment team does not know your loved one as well as you do, your input may be invaluable, especially if the resident is not able to provide meaningful input. Although development of a care plan is something required to be done by a nursing home, a care plan can, and ideally should, be created in advance, well before the need for nursing home care. By planning in advance, when you have a clear mind and the ability to communicate effectively, you can much better guarantee that your wishes, lifestyles and desires are documented and will be communicated to your future caregivers, whether these be family members, private nurses, home health aides, or staff in a nursing home.

The easiest way to develop your own care plan is to use a tool such as the Advance Care Plan, created by Advance Care Planning, Inc. The Advance Care Plan is a proprietary document that is created by special software that gathers, organizes, stores and disseminates information provided by you in an interview, in order to better serve your future healthcare needs and to guide those who you will depend or for future care. The Advance Care Plan identifies your specific needs, desires, habits and preferences and guides your caregiver in a unique manner. An Advance Care Plan should be created as part of your basic Estate Plan or as part of your Long-Term Care Plan, because the best person to create a care plan for you is you. The following example is provided by Advance Care Planning, Inc. of how an Advance Care Plan can help improve a day in the life of Lynn, a typical nursing home resident:

Lynn, at the age of 85, has been placed in the nursing home due to a stroke. She is incontinent, but if taken to the restroom at appropriate times she will be continent most of the time. She is alert, but somewhat confused at times. She very much knows what she wants but cannot always verbalize it. She is able to feed herself finger foods.

Without an Advance Care Plan	**With an Advance Care Plan**
5:30 AM: Awakened. Hospital gown taken off, given some quick care, dressed for the day in someone else's house dress. It is a pretty house dress, but she does not like house dresses.	7:00 AM: Awakened. Taken to the bathroom for quick morning care, then placed in a comfortable chair in her room in front of the TV with a requested show on to await breakfast. Stays in her short PJ's and a robe since it is a shower day.
7:30AM: Taken to the dining room for breakfast. Given one cup of coffee, not offered more coffee. Not served bacon due to her high cholesterol.	7:30AM: Served bacon and eggs for breakfast. Her cholesterol is high, but she stated her wishes to eat a regular diet, including bacon and eggs for breakfast, in her Advance Care Plan. She has two cups of coffee, as she has done for the last 65 years.

After Breakfast: Taken to sit in the hallway outside of her room.	After Breakfast: Taken to the bathroom and then to shower room. Her hair is washed, as it is with every shower per her Advance Care Plan. She prefers to shower in the morning. After shower, dressed in her navy blue jogging suit with her red tee shirt, per her Advance Care Plan.
1-2 hours Later: Taken to her room, has her brief changed and then is set in the hallway by the nurse's station. Her lips were not moistened, nor does she have access to chapstick.	1-2 Hours Later: Has her chapstick around her neck and is able to put it on herself frequently. Though her lips do not look dry, they feel dry to her. Her Advance Care Plan notes that the staff should help her moisten her lips frequently.
10:00 AM: Given six pills – two for high cholesterol, one for irregular heartbeat, one for hiatal hernia to prevent heart burn, one for hypertension and one for arthritis.	10:00 AM: Given three pills – one for hiatal hernia to prevent heartburn, one for hypertension and one for arthritis. Decided in her Advance Care Plan that if she ever entered a nursing home she would prefer not to take the other medications.

11:00 AM: Still sitting in the hall by the nurse's station.	11:00 AM: Taken outside to sit in the shade. She does not like crafts, but prefers to be outside in the shade, weather permitting.
12:00 Noon: Taken to the dining room for lunch. Given a lean hamburger, no salt allowed, a salad with lowfat dressing and applesauce. Needs assistance with the applesauce.	12:00 Noon: Taken back to her room for lunch; placed in her chair in front of the TV with her program of choice. Given a cheeseburger, packets of salt, french fries and apple slices. Her Advance Care Plan states that she does not want to be spoon-fed and would prefer finger foods.
After Lunch: Taken to the nurse's station to sit in the hallway.	After Lunch: Taken to the restroom and then placed in her recliner to rest and watch her favorite movie on her DVD player.
2:00 PM: Placed in bed to have brief changed, and rest.	2:00 PM: Still watching her movie.
3:30 PM: Placed in wheelchair and taken to ceramics class.	3:30 PM: Gets her weekly manicure instead of going to ceramics class. She does not like crafts.
5:00 PM: Taken to room to have brief changed.	5:00 PM: Taken to the restroom. Prepared for dinner.

5:30 PM: Taken to dining room for dinner. Served chicken. Lynn loves hot dogs but they are not served to her due to her high cholesterol.	5:30 PM: Placed in her chair in her room for dinner. Served hot dogs with green pepper slices, cherry tomatoes and veggie dip. Enjoyed a brownie for dessert.
After Dinner: Taken to the nurse's station to sit in the hall. There is a TV with DVD at the nurse's station; staff puts a movie on for those sitting in the hall to watch. The movie is one which Lynn has seen several times and does not like.	After Dinner: She continues to watch TV until 7:30 PM.
8:30 PM: Taken to the shower. She prefers to bathe in the morning.	7:30 PM: Taken to the bathroom and helped to prepare for bed. She wears her short pajamas per her Advance Care Plan.
After Shower: Dressed in a hospital gown and put to bed with one pillow at her head.	8:00 PM: Placed in bed with a talking book. It is a legal mystery, the type of book she likes. She has stated in her Advance Care Plan that she likes to go to bed by 8:00 PM to read. She is only able to make use of talking books at this time.

The room is 75 degrees and she is very warm. She throws her covers off since she is too warm to sleep. The staff does come in and turn her several times. They place her on her back (she has never been able to sleep on her back) and they always cover her back up. Her brief is changed once during the night.	In bed, she has down pillows (5 ft.) on either side of her, between her legs, and 3 at her head, as she has slept for 40 years. The room temperature is 70 degrees, which is slightly warm for her. The temperature cannot be adjusted due to her roommate, so her personal fan is turned on to keep her cooler. She sleeps well but is awakened by the staff twice to take her to the toilet, per her Advance Care Plan. She remains continent at night.
The following day, she falls asleep in her chair by the nurse's station since she did not sleep well the night before. Her children come to take her out to lunch but she appears too sleepy so she does not go.	The following day she is rested and has a strong sense of well-being. Her children come and take her to lunch. She is gone several hours, and rests in her chair for two hours upon her return.

If you have not created an Advance Care Plan prior to entering a nursing home, the assessment team at the nursing home will gather information from your friends and family members to develop a care plan. The formal care plan defines specific care the resident needs and outlines strategies the staff will use to meet them. The assessment team meets during the first month of a new resident's placement at a care planning meeting. Family members, as well as the resident, may attend. When you go to the care plan meeting, bring along a copy of the list of needs you gave the assessment team earlier. Together, you can discuss your loved one's needs and the care plan the team has developed. If some need has been overlooked, you can ensure that the assessment team addresses it during this meeting.

The formal care plan becomes part of the nursing home contract. It should detail the resident's medical, emotional and social needs and spell out what will be done to improve (when possible) or maintain the resident's health.

Federal law requires that nursing home care result in improvement if improvement is possible. In cases where improvement is not possible, the care must maintain abilities or slow the loss of function. For example, if your mother has a slight problem with language when she moves into the nursing home, the care plan should include activities that encourage her use of language unless or until the disease's progression changes this ability.

Federal law also requires that nursing homes review the resident's care plan every three months and whenever the resident's condition changes. It must also reassess the resident annually. For example, if your father had bladder control when he entered the nursing home, but has since become incontinent, this significant change in his status means the nursing home staff must develop a new care plan that addresses his new need.

As a care advocate, you'll want to monitor your loved one's care to be sure the nursing home is providing the care outlined in the care plan. You should also attend all care planning meetings, whether regularly scheduled or when held because of a change in your loved one's health. By being as involved as possible with the care planning process, you will help to ensure that your loved one gets the best possible care while in the nursing home.

chapter 9

THE RIGHTS OF NURSING HOME RESIDENTS

Residents of nursing homes enjoy the same constitutional and civil rights they had when they were living in their own homes. In fact, residents are protected by state and federal laws which recognize their vulnerability. Residents and family members should become familiar with these laws to make certain their rights are being protected.

All nursing homes that accept Medicare or Medicaid are required to comply with the Nursing Home Reform Act.[3] This law was enacted to ensure that nursing home residents "attain or maintain the highest practicable physical, mental and psychosocial well-being." In addition to this federal act, Virginia has its own set of regulations governing the rights of nursing home residents and residents of assisted living facilities.[4] Taken together, the federal Nursing Home Reform Act and Virginia's statutes provide a sweeping "Bill of Rights" for all residents of nursing homes and assisted living facilities, whether receiving federal funds or private-pay. The following is a summary of these important protections.

---

[3] The Nursing Home Reform Act, part of the Omnibus Budget Reconciliation Act of 1987.

[4] Virginia Code § 32.1-138 and § 63.2-1808. These regulations also apply to continuing care retirement communities that offer nursing care or assisting living for residents within their facility.

THE RIGHT TO MAKE DECISIONS

Nursing home residents may exercise their rights as citizens without interference from the nursing home. Nursing home residents have the right to make financial and medical decisions -- including the right to check out of the nursing home — unless the resident has chosen, in advance, who will assert his or her rights if the resident is no longer able to do so (via a financial and/or health care power of attorney) or if a court has appointed someone to make those decisions (guardianship/conservatorship).

THE RIGHT TO BE FULLY INFORMED

Upon admission to a facility, a residents is entitled to information about the rights of residents of the facility. Each resident must be informed orally and in writing of those rights. Residents have the right to be informed of the services offered and charges for those services (including those not covered by the facility's daily rate); residents are entitled to know the facility's regulations, the results of state inspections, the procedures for transfer, and the names and addresses of every owner of the facility.

Residents have the right to be informed of their medical condition and treatment plan. Residents have the right to receive notice of changes concerning their treatment, including but not limited to altering medications, a change in physical or mental status, room or roommate changes, and a transfer or discharge from the nursing home. In addition, if a nursing home changes its charges or services, it is required to notify the residents, in writing, at least 30 days before the change goes into effect.

THE RIGHT TO PARTICIPATE IN CARE PLANNING

Residents have the right to full participation in their care planning — including the right to refuse services and the right to refuse medical treatment. Residents have the right to participate in their own care plan meetings (and invite anyone they wish to attend those meetings, as well). Residents must be able to choose their own doctor and choose a pharmacy (so long as the pharmacy's unit dose system is the same as the nursing home's). Unless the attending physician or interdisciplinary team has determined it unsafe, each resident has the right to self-administer his or her medications.

Residents have the right to inspect their charts and may, upon written request, obtain copies of all of their own records. Residents have the right to information regarding how to examine those records, as well.

THE RIGHT TO BE TREATED WITH DIGNITY AND RESPECT

One of the most fundamental rights, and also one of the most overlooked, is the legal right residents have to be treated with dignity and respect. So long as it is not detrimental to their care plan, residents have the right to make their own schedules and choose which activities they attend. In making their own schedules, residents have the right to decide what time they wake up in the morning, what time they eat their meals and what time they go to bed at night.

Residents have the right to be addressed in the manner they choose — whether by a formal title — such as Mr. Smith, Mrs. Jones, Dr. Baker or General Johnson — or by a first name or a nickname if that is their preference.

The Right To Confidentiality

All information regarding personal, financial, medical and social affairs is privileged and is to be kept confidential. The nursing home may not show the resident's chart to other people or agencies without permission, nor may they discuss treatment options with others unless they have permission.

The Right To Privacy

Residents have the right to privacy in all aspects of life. They have the right to meet privately with any visitors (family, friends, physician, ombudsman, legal representative or anyone else), to send and receive private, unopened mail, and to make private telephone calls. Residents have the right to have all medical and personal care provided with privacy, using visual barriers to prevent others from viewing care and treatment. Residents have the right to perform all bodily functions (bathing, toileting, etc.) in private. If assistance is required, only those staff members needed to help should be present. Subject to possible restrictions based on care needs or payor source, residents have the right to take trips out of the facility for lunch or dinner, for a family holiday, or for a weekend visit.

The Right to Voice Grievances

Every nursing home must have a system to address concerns relating to residents' treatment or care. This includes grievances residents have concerning the behavior of other residents. Residents have the right to prompt efforts for resolution by the nursing home. The staff and administration are prohibited by law from retaliation for complaints. The nursing home must also post information relating to pertinent government and advocacy organizations (such as the number and address for the Long Term Care Ombudsman). Residents, of course, maintain the right to report crimes to the local police and/or district attorney.

THE RIGHT TO MANAGE FINANCES

Residents have the right to manage their own financial affairs. Residents cannot be required to deposit personal funds with the nursing home. If the residents choose to deposit funds with the nursing home, the facility must manage the residents' funds properly. Residents have the right to written quarterly accountings of their funds.

THE RIGHT TO KEEP PERSONAL PROPERTY AND HAVE IT SECURED

All nursing homes are required to have a written policy concerning protection of residents' personal property. If a resident's property is lost, and the nursing home is responsible for the loss, the resident may have a claim against the nursing home to replace the property.

THE RIGHT TO BE FREE FROM ABUSE AND NEGLECT

Residents have the right to be free from physical, sexual, verbal, and mental abuse. Residents have the right to be free from corporal punishment and involuntary seclusion. Residents have the right to be free from neglect. Any failure by the nursing home to provide the resident with necessary services, including those identified in the resident's care plan, constitutes neglect and is a violation of residents' rights. Residents have the right to express complaints and concerns without fear of retaliation.

THE RIGHT TO BE FREE FROM PHYSICAL AND CHEMICAL RESTRAINTS

Residents have the right to be free from unnecessary physical restraints (vest restraints, hand mitts, four point restraints and any and all other physical restraints) and unnecessary chemical restraints (anti-psychotic drugs, sedatives, and any and all other chemical restraints). Restraints are to be used only as treatment for medical symptoms and must be prescribed by a physician. Chemical or physical restraints are not to be used for disciplinary measures, nor may they be used for staff convenience.

The Right Against Unlawful Discharge Or Transfer And The Right To Re-Admission

Due to the seriousness of discharging a resident (the transfer trauma suffered by the resident, the stress undergone by the family members locating a new facility, etc.), the regulations concerning unlawful discharge are very specific and must be followed precisely. A nursing facility may only discharge a resident for the following reasons:

- It can no longer meet the resident's medical needs as documented in writing by the resident's own physician;
- Non-payment after reasonable notice; or
- The resident is a danger to self or others, as documented by the physician (if relating to a health issue) or as documented by the nursing home (if relating to patients' safety).

Unless it is an emergency situation, residents must be given written notice 30 days prior to the date of discharge. The "discharge notice" must state the reason for the discharge and the location to which the resident is to be transferred or discharged. The notice must also provide information regarding the right to appeal the discharge.

If a resident is transferred or discharged, the nursing home must develop a discharge plan which provides comprehensive information allowing for continuity of care in the resident's new home.

If a resident requires intermittent hospitalization or therapy outside of the nursing home, for whatever reason, the nursing home must provide the resident with a written copy of its bed hold policy. Specifically, the nursing home must inform the resident how long it will hold the bed and how much the bed hold will cost.

chapter 10
Recognizing Abuse & Neglect

There are several different types of abuse, some of which are more obvious than others. The following are the types of abuse or violation of rights that often occur. We've also included the signs to look for.

Types Of Physical Abuse

Physical abuse is perhaps the most obvious, and is usually easier to detect than other forms of abuse. The most common types of physical abuse are:

- Assault — hitting, shaking, pushing, shoving, kicking, burning, choking, scratching, rough-handling, cutting, biting, physically confining, forcibly confining or restraining into a room, a chair, a bed;
- Forcibly feeding;
- Forcibly medicating;
- Over-medicating;
- Sexually molesting;
- Any sexual activity with an adult who is unable to understand or give consent;
- Inflicting pornography, voyeurism, exhibitionism, etc.;
- Control of an adult through the use of threats or intimidation or through the abuse of a relationship of trust;

- Prolonged intervals between an injury and the treatment;
- Frequent changes in doctors.

Signs of Physical Abuse

The most common signs of physical abuse are:

- Cuts, scrapes, burns, puncture wounds, marks indicating use of restraints.
- Bruises, discoloration, swelling.
- Difficulty moving.
- Stiffness (trouble walking or sitting). The resident may have been injured internally or suffered broken bones with no external signs.
- Genital infections or pain in the groin area.

Ask the resident what happened. Do they have an explanation for the injury? Is it believable, or do the injuries lead you to a different conclusion?

Types Of Psychological Abuse

There are varying degrees of psychological / emotional abuse. Often, this type of abuse is difficult to detect, particularly if you do not witness interactions between the abuser and the resident. The most common types of psychological abuse are:

- Threatening residents (threatening to physically harm residents, threatening to take away their rights, threatening to sell their property, threatening to place them in confinement, threatening to take the residents' power to make choices, etc.);
- Humiliating residents or treating them like children;

- Verbal abuse, insults, name calling;

Signs Of Psychological Abuse

The most common signs of psychological abuse are:

- Helplessness;
- Hesitation to talk openly;
- Agitation and/or trouble sleeping;
- Withdrawal and/or depression;
- Implausible stories;
- Fear in the presence of the caregiver;
- Constant deferral to the caregiver, including waiting for the caregiver to answer a question which was posed to the resident;
- Decision-making by the caregiver without deferring or consulting with the resident;
- Resident not accepting/allowing visitors.

Types Of Neglect

Whether intentional or unintentional, any time residents are left in an unsafe environment or they are not receiving proper care, they are being neglected. The most common types of neglect are:

- Withholding treatment (failing to administer medications, failing to provide physical therapy when needed, not taking to doctor's appointments, etc.);
- Failing to provide assistance with Activities of Daily Living (e.g., toileting, bathing, transferring, eating, etc.), when necessary;
- Withholding food;

- Failing to ensure proper diet;
- Abandoning the resident;
- Failing to provide basic needs - food, clothing, shelter, medicine, medical aids not properly or timely administered.

Signs Of Neglect

The most common signs of neglect are:

- Malnourishment;
- Dehydration;
- Weight loss;
- Not receiving proper medical care (under or over medicated, missing doctor's appointments, etc.);
- Lacking necessary medical aids (walker, wheelchair, hearing aid, dentures, etc.);
- The presence of pressure sores;
- Inadequate personal hygiene;
- Inadequate and/or inappropriate clothing;
- Inadequate and/or inappropriate supervision;
- Extreme filth of person or surrounding;
- Pest/rodent infestation;
- Offensive odors;
- Inadequate heat, fuel, electricity, refrigeration;
- Untreated physical or mental health problems;
- Abandonment;

- Dilapidated housing condition;
- Soiled bedding.

Types Of Financial Abuse

Financial abuse, technically called "exploitation," is common among residents and takes on many different forms. Often caregivers coerce residents into selling their property, or giving or loaning them money. Caregivers may obtain the same results through fraud, forgery, and through the crimes of larceny, embezzlement, theft by false pretenses, burglary, false impersonation, and extortion. The most common types of financial abuse are:

- Withholding money belonging to the resident;
- Forcing a resident to sell or give property away;
- Stealing money from a resident;
- Coercing a resident to give away money;
- Borrowing money from a resident and failing to repay it.

Signs Of Financial Abuse

The most common signs of financial abuse are:

- The resident cannot explain the disappearance of funds in bank account;
- The resident's personal property is missing and he/she has no explanation;
- The resident is suddenly spending a great deal of money;
- The resident suddenly withdraws a lot of money from accounts;

- The resident is unable to pay his or her bills;
- The caregiver does not give the resident an opportunity to speak for him or herself;
- The caregiver is defensive;
- The caregiver gives conflicting accounts of incidents reported by the others (i.e. incidents reported by the resident, family members, friends, neighbors, other health care professionals);
- The caregiver has drug or alcohol problems;
- The caregiver has history of past abuse;
- The caregiver's affection is inappropriate (flirtations, coyness, or other indications that there may be an inappropriate sexual relationship).

chapter 11

Protection From Abuse and Neglect

Often residents are not aware they are being abused, perhaps because it has gone on for so long they don't consider it abuse, or perhaps because they suffer a mental illness which renders them incapable of recognizing abuse. Therefore, it is extremely important to be aware of their situation and note any changes that occur. The following are some things that you can do on an ongoing basis to protect the resident.

Stay Informed

The resident's health may change, the staffing and administration may change, policies may change, etc. Talk regularly with the resident and establish a relationship with the resident which allows the resident to trust you. Don't ever dismiss what the resident tells you simply because the resident has dementia or some other mental illness which in your mind renders him or her "incompetent."

Educate And Empower Both Yourself And The Resident

Utilize your resources. Resident and Family Councils, for example, are great sources of information inside the nursing home. Outside the nursing home, the Long Term Care Ombudsman is a great resource for advocates. Adult Protective Services is not only reactive, but is a preventive and supportive agency with a wealth of information. Your local Area Agency on Aging is another state agency which provides helpful information, as do outside organizations like the American Association of Retired Persons (AARP) and support groups sponsored by such organizations as the

Alzheimer's Association. In today's world, the Internet is also a vast resource for all kinds of educational information relating to the rights of the elderly. Be sure to share information with the resident whenever possible. Keep in mind that the more control residents have over their lives, the fewer opportunities abusers have to take advantage of them.

Establish Relationships

Establish relationships with the nursing home staff and with the other residents and their family members. The nursing home staff are with your loved one 24 hours a day. Get to know them. They can be your "eyes and ears" and alert you to possible abuse. Establish a relationship that is both professional and friendly. Do not speak with them only when you are expressing concern or dissatisfaction. Be sure to let them know what you are pleased with.

Other residents and their family members can be both a great support system and a significant source of information. All nursing homes are required to facilitate Resident and Family Councils. These monthly meetings of residents and family members are a way to help one another address shared concerns.

Take An Active Role In The Resident's Care Planning

Attend the monthly care plan meetings (also encourage the resident to attend whenever possible). If the resident has special needs that you are aware of, be sure to let the interdisciplinary team know. Suggest a few ways the resident's needs can be met. Don't be afraid to ask questions. Make sure you understand and agree with the care plan. Obtain a copy of the plan and be sure to follow up with the staff to ensure the care plan is being met.

If you have permission from the resident, periodically review the resident's charts. The first few times you review the chart, ask a staff member to review the chart with you and explain those sections which are confusing to you. Periodically review the resident's financial records, as well (provided the resident has given you permission). Make a list of the residents's personal belongings and periodically check to make sure that all belongings remain accounted for. Many residents also label their belongings for easy identification.

Document Your Concerns

When you visit the resident, keep a journal. Record your observations and keep track of patterns. Note statements made by witnesses. Be sure you record dates and times. Take photographs and videos. When reporting incidents, it helps to have clearly-defined symptoms and conditions. Accuracy is important. If you should ever need to file a complaint, detailed records enable outside parties to have an accurate description of events.

chapter 12
IF YOU SUSPECT ABUSE OR NEGLECT

If you suspect a nursing home resident is being neglected or abused and the situation requires immediate action, you should speak with the Director of Nursing or the Administrator of the nursing home. You should also report the incident to the Virginia Elder Abuse Hotline. Every state has an Elder Abuse Hotline that takes calls from concerned persons who suspect abuse of residents (both domestic and institutional). In Virginia, the Elder Abuse Hotline is 1-888-832-3858 (in-state only). If you are out of state, you must call 804-371-0896. This Hotline is available 24 hours, 7 days a week, 365 days a year. Additionally, all health care workers or nursing home employees who have reason to suspect that an adult has been abused, neglected, or exploited are required to immediately report the incident to the local office of Adult Protective Services.

Problems which are not emergencies and do not rise to the level of abuse or neglect are best resolved at the least formal level. If it is a non-emergency, first speak with the staff person(s) whose job is related to your concern. When you are discussing the problem, cite specific examples. If you are not satisfied with the response, contact the supervisor, the Director of Nursing, or the Administrator of the nursing home. Don't automatically defer to the nursing home employees or assume they are acting within the confines of the law. If a nursing facility staff member tells you "that's the law," demand to know exactly which law he or she means. Similarly, don't automatically defer to a staff member who tells you "these types of things happen," or "nothing can be done." Each facility has a Rights Advisor whose job is to field complaints. Put your concern in writing. The Rights Advisor is required to provide a written response within 30 days of receiving the complaint. If you are not satisfied with the response of the Rights Advisor, your next step is to speak with a Long Term Care Ombudsman. The Long Term Care Ombudsman Program, established in all states under the Older Americans Act, is authorized to investigate and resolve complaints on behalf of nursing home residents. Ombudsmen advocate on behalf of residents and work to bring about changes on local, state, and national levels to ensure quality care.

In addition to state offices responsible for investigating abuse, Virginia also has three private citizen advocacy groups for the elderly, which are listed in **Appendix D** (page 142).

If you are still not satisfied with the results you have received, or if the abuse is of such a grave nature that you feel the nursing home has violated the law, consult an elder law attorney. If an injury or other violation of the law has occurred, an elder law attorney can advise you as to whether there are potential legal actions that you may be able to successfully pursue.

chapter 13

Estate Planning and Powers of Attorney

We all know that we will eventually die. At the same time, no one likes to dwell on the prospect of his or her own death. But if you, your parents, or other loved ones postpone planning until it is too late, you run the risk that your children or other intended beneficiaries — those you love the most — may not receive all that you would hope, or may not be taken care of in the way you would hope. That is what estate planning is all about — making sure that your loved ones are taken care of when you are gone. All adults need to do estate planning — whether you have fifty thousand or five million dollars, you probably want to distribute your assets in a certain way upon your death, which means you need to do estate planning.

We should begin a discussion of estate planning with a review of what "estate" and "estate plan" mean.

An "estate" is everything you own: bank accounts, stocks and bonds, real estate, motor vehicles, retirement plans, life insurance, jewelry, household furniture, etc.

An "estate plan," generally, refers to the means by which your estate is passed on to your loved ones on your death. Estate planning can be accomplished through a variety of methods, including:

- Revocable Living Trusts
- Last Will and Testament / Probate
- Lifetime Gifting

- Joint Ownership
- Beneficiary Designations
- Life Estates

Problems often arise when people don't coordinate all of these methods of passing on their estate. To take just one example, a father's will may say that everything should be equally divided among his children, but if the father creates a joint account with only one of the children "for the sake of convenience," there could be a fight about whether that account should be put back in the pool with the rest of the property.

A well-crafted estate plan permits your family to save potentially hundreds of thousands of dollars on taxes, court costs and attorneys' fees. Most importantly, it affords the comfort that your loved ones can mourn your loss without being simultaneously burdened with unnecessary red tape and financial confusion.

Good estate planning also includes signing three additional documents: (1) an Advance Medical Directive, which includes a Living Will and a Medical Power of Attorney; (2) a Durable General Power of Attorney for legal and financial affairs; and (3) an Advance Care Plan. Taken together, these three important documents allow you to decide in advance who will manage your legal, personal, and financial affairs in the event of your disability, and exactly how you will be cared for. Estate planning (including the decision as to whether to use a Will or a Living Trust as your primary estate planning tool), is vitally important for someone who may soon be entering a nursing home.

Because most people use a Revocable Living Trust as their primary estate planning tool, a basic understanding of Living Trusts is important when planning your estate. Since the purpose of a Living Trust is to avoid probate, to understand the usefulness of a Living Trust you must first understand how probate works.

EXPLANATION OF PROBATE

Using a Last Will and Testament as your primary estate planning tool means that your estate will go through probate upon your death. Although the probate process is quite complicated and time-consuming for the executor, the purpose of probate is to provide some measure of protection for your beneficiaries.

Phase 1 of Probate: To initiate the probate process in Virginia, an Executor nominated in a Last Will and Testament must take the original Will and an original death certificate and make at least one appearance at the probate office to officially "qualify" and be "sworn in" as executor. Once qualified, an executor is accountable to the probate court and is required to prepare and file various legal and financial documents, including a detailed initial inventory of the estate and detailed annual accountings showing everything coming in to and going out of the estate. During the initial phase of probate, the executor must see to it that all estate assets are accounted for and that any valid debts, expenses, and taxes are paid. There are strict limitations during this initial probate phase as to how much the executor may distribute as support to a surviving spouse and/or minor children. After at least one year from the date of death (and often significantly longer), the Executor may distribute the remaining assets of the estate either:

1. To the beneficiaries you have named;
2. To the trustee named in your Will (if your Will has testamentary trust provisions, typically because your beneficiaries are under a specified age), to be held and administered according to the testamentary trust provisions set forth in your Will and subject to ongoing probate; or
3. To the trustee named in your Living Trust (if you have a Living Trust) to be held outside of probate and administered

according to the terms set forth in your Living Trust, free of any court supervision.

Phase 2 of Probate: If your Will has provisions for the creation of a testamentary trust upon the conclusion of the initial phase of probate, then the testamentary trustee named in your Will is accountable to the probate court and, just like the executor, is required to prepare and file various legal and financial documents, including a detailed initial inventory of the trust and detailed accountings showing everything coming in to and going out of the trust every year. During this second phase of probate, the trustee must see to it that all trust assets are accounted for and that any valid debts, expenses, and taxes are paid from the trust when due. Upon the occurrence of a pre-determined event (typically a beneficiary reaching a specified age), the trustee may then terminate the trust by distributing all remaining assets to your named beneficiaries.

Explanation of Revocable Living Trusts

A trust is a legal entity which is capable of owning financial assets, real estate, and/or other property.

A testamentary trust, as explained above, is a trust created by the Probate Court pursuant to trust provisions written into your Last Will and Testament. A testamentary trust does not take effect until after your death and generally not until after your Executor has completed the initial phase of probate. Trustees of testamentary trusts in Virginia are generally required to file accountings with the Commissioner of Accounts every year that the trust exists.

A **living trust** is a trust that comes into existence during your lifetime, and a Revocable Living Trust is simply a living trust that can be revoked or modified during your lifetime, as opposed to some living trusts that are irrevocable. Using a Revocable Living Trust as your primary estate planning tool means that your estate will not go through probate upon your death. You create a Revocable Living Trust by signing a contractual document called a "Declaration of Trust" or "Trust Agreement." You are typically the trustee of your own trust until your death, although if you are about to enter a nursing home you may decide to make someone else your initial trustee. If you are the initial trustee, then upon your death, a successor trustee whom you have named takes over as trustee of the trust and, after paying any valid debts, expenses, and taxes, distributes the trust assets to or for the benefit of your named beneficiaries or, if called for in the trust, continues to hold the trust assets until the occurrence of a predetermined event.

The main feature of a Revocable Living Trust is that the trustee is not accountable to the court, and therefore not subject to probate. Most people therefore use a Revocable Living Trust as their primary estate planning tool in order to make things easier for their trusted loved ones by avoiding the time and complications of probate. There may also be some advantages to you by using a Revocable Living Trust to consolidate your assets and simplify your finances. On the other hand, some people like the idea of court supervision and therefore prefer that their estate go through probate, and some people simply prefer not to spend the extra money it typically takes to create a living trust or the extra time it takes to properly fund a living trust.

Financial Power of Attorney

A Durable General Financial Power of Attorney authorizes your agent, called "Attorney-in-Fact," to act on your behalf and sign your name to financial and/or legal documents. The Financial Power of Attorney is an essential tool if you are unable to carry on your legal and financial affairs due to age, illness, or injury. Having a Financial Power of Attorney will generally avoid the need to go through the time-consuming, expensive, and publicly embarrassing guardianship process, which process is subject to probate court supervision. During the guardianship process, someone goes to court to have you declared mentally or physically incompetent and the court appoints one or more persons to serve as your legal guardian and/or conservator.

Health Care Power of Attorney

A Health Care Power of Attorney (also called a Medical Power of Attorney or an Advance Medical Directive) authorizes another person (called your "Medical Agent"), to make decisions with respect to your medical care in the event that you are physically or mentally unable to do so, as certified by two physicians. This document includes the type of provisions that used to be in what was commonly called a "Living Will," allowing you to indicate your wishes concerning the use of artificial or extraordinary measures to prolong your life artificially in the event of a terminal illness or injury. You will also use this document to indicate your wishes with regard to organ donation, disposition of bodily remains, and funeral arrangements.

Advance Care Plan

An Advance Care Plan is a document that is created by special software that gathers, organizes, stores and disseminates information provided by you in an interview, in order to better serve your future healthcare needs and to guide those who you will depend or for future care. The Advance Care Plan identifies your specific needs, desires, habits and preferences and guides your caregiver in a unique manner. See page 57 for a detailed example of the tremendous benefits of an Advance Care Plan.

chapter 14
LEGAL ASSISTANCE

Aging persons and their family members face many unique legal issues. As you have read in this book, the Medicaid program and the myriad legal, financial, care planning, and estate planning issues facing the prospective nursing home resident and family can be particularly complex. If you or a family member needs nursing home care, it is clear that you need expert legal help. Where can you turn for that help? It is difficult for the consumer to identify lawyers who have the training and experience required to provide expert guidance during this most difficult time.

Nursing home planning, Medicaid planning, asset protection planning, and estate planning are all services provided by elder law attorneys. Consumers must be cautious in choosing a lawyer and should always carefully investigate the lawyer's credentials.

The most important and most widely-recognized credential in the field of elder law is the CELA (Certified Elder Law Attorney) designation. The CELA designation is administered by the Board of Certification of the National Elder Law Foundation, which is the only organization accredited by the American Bar Association to certify lawyers in the specialty area of elder law. Among the numerous criteria required for certification, CELAs must pass a rigorous full-day certification examination and receive favorable peer reviews from at least five other attorneys familiar with their competence and qualifications in elder law. CELAs also must have, during the three years prior to certification: handled at least 60 elder law matters with a specified distribution among 12 different areas of elder law and participated in at least 45 hours of continuing legal education in elder law. You can locate a CELA in your area by visiting www.nelf.org.

The leading professional organization of elder law attorneys is NAELA — the National Academy of Elder Law Attorneys — which also has a Virginia Chapter. Though mere membership in the Academy is open to any lawyer and is no guarantee that the attorney is experienced in elder law, membership does at least show that the lawyer has a genuine interest in the field. In addition, NAELA runs several educational sessions each year as well as an Internet discussion group to help attorney members stay current on the latest aspects of elder law. You can find a listing of NAELA members in your area by visiting www.naela.org, which will also tell you if the attorney is a Certified Elder Law Attorney.

According to NAELA, the other top three organizations you may want to call for lawyer referrals are: your local chapter of the Alzheimer's Association or AARP (see **Appendix B**, page 129), or your local Area Agency on Aging (see **Appendix C**, page 134). NAELA suggests you ask lots of questions before selecting an elder law attorney, as you don't want to end up in the office of an attorney who can't help you. Start with the initial phone call. It is not unusual to speak only to a secretary or receptionist during an initial call; however, many elder law attorneys do offer free initial phone consultations to determine if your issue is something they can help you with. NAELA suggests asking the following questions during your first call: How long has the attorney been in practice? Does his/her practice emphasize a particular area of law? How long has he/she been in this field? What percentage of his/her practice is devoted to elder law? Is there a fee for the first consultation and if so, how much? Given the nature of your problem, what information should you bring with you to the initial consultation?

The answers to your questions will assist you in determining whether that particular attorney has those qualifications important to you for a successful attorney/client relationship. If you have a specific legal issue that requires immediate attention, be sure to inform the office of this during the initial telephone conversation.

In addition to looking for attorneys with the CELA designation and who are members of NAELA, you may want to seek recommendations from any friends and family members who have received professional help with elder law and/or nursing home issues (who did they use and were they satisfied with the services they received?). Hospital social workers, discharge planners, accountants, financial professionals, and even other attorneys can also be good sources of recommendations.

Most states and many local bar associations have formal lawyer referral services that can refer you to an elder law attorney. Be aware, however, that many bar association referral services allow new or inexperienced attorneys to join and do not limit the number of attorneys who may join, so if you use a referral service be sure to check how it operates.

The Internet can be another good source of information about elder law attorneys. The most sell-known service that offers independent ratings of attorneys by their peers is Martindale-Hubbell Law Directory, at www.martindale.com. Look for attorneys who are rated AV or BV, which indicates professional standards of conduct and ethics, reliability, diligence, an exemplary reputation, and a well-established practice. You can also find out a lot about an attorney from his or her own Web site — most attorneys these days have Web sites that list at least their educational background and the types of cases they handle — many attorneys have much larger Web sites that provide valuable free information, helpful forms, and even offer a way to obtain legal advice online or via email if you are so inclined. A good example is www.VirginiaElderLaw.com.

In general, a lawyer who devotes a substantial part of his or her practice to elder law and nursing home planning should have more knowledge and experience to address the issues properly. Don't hesitate to ask the lawyer what percentage of his practice involves nursing home planning. Or you may want to ask how many new nursing home planning cases the law office handles each month. There is no correct answer. But there is a good chance that a law office that assists with one or two nursing home placements a week is likely to be more up-to-date and knowledgeable than an office that helps with one or two placements a year.

Ask whether the lawyer is involved with committees or local or state bar organizations that have to do with elder law or estate planning? If so, has the lawyer held a position of authority on the committee? Does the lawyer lecture on elder law and/or estate planning? If so, to whom? If the lawyer lectures to the public, you might try to attend one of the seminars. This should help you decide if this lawyer is right for you. If the lawyer is asked to speak at educational seminars to other lawyers about elder law and nursing home planning, that is a very good sign that the lawyer is considered to be knowledgeable by people who ought to know.

Another leading organization that some elder law attorneys are affiliated with is NAFEP— the National Association of Financial and Estate Planning (www.nafep.org) which offers the Certified Estate Advisor designation. Certified Estate Advisors have special expertise in many complex financial and estate planning strategies. Attorneys who are Certified Estate Advisors are also able to offer a complete range of estate planning services for every person's estate.

In the end, follow your instincts and choose an attorney who knows this area of the law, who is committed to helping others, and who will listen to you and the unique desires and needs of you and your family.

CONCLUSION

As you have sees, there are numerous strategies that you can use to qualify for Medicaid and still preserve — for yourself and, if desired, for your children or other heirs — some or all of the assets you've spent a lifetime building.

These strategies are legal. They are moral. They are ethical. Medicaid planning is no different from income tax planning (trying to find all of the proper and legal deductions that you are entitled to) or estate tax planning (trying to plan your estate to minimize the amount of estate tax that will be paid). However, as this book has explained numerous times, Medicaid planning requires a great deal of extremely complicated knowledge about the Medicaid system and its complex regulations. You need to work with an experienced legal advisor who knows the rules and can advise you properly.

In the previous pages, we've talked about how to find the right nursing home, how to get good care there, and how to pay for it without going broke. Where do you actually start looking? The easiest place to start is on the next page — **Appendix A** — a listing of all nursing homes in Virginia organized by region. If placement is not urgent, telephone each nursing facility in your nearby area and ask for its information packet, including an activity calendar and a menu. Next, if you have Internet access, go to NHCompare, Medicare's Nursing Home Comparison Website at www.medicare.gov/NHCompare. Next, browse through the resources listed in **Appendix B** (page 129) and **Appendix C** (page 134).

Once you've determined which facilities you want to tour, then you can use the Evaluation Tool on page 14 to help you compare them.

Good luck to you and your family as you embark on this challenging journey of transition.

APPENDIX A — VIRGINIA NURSING HOMES ORGANIZED BY REGION

NORTHERN VIRGINIA NURSING HOMES

Annaburg Manor 9201 Maple St Manassas, VA 20110 (703) 335-8300
Birmingham Green 8605 Centreville Rd Manassas, VA 20110 (703) 257-0935
Burke HealthCare Center 9640 Burke Lake Rd Burke, VA 22015 (703) 425-9765
Cherrydale Health & Rehab Center 3710 Lee Hwy Arlington, VA 22207 (703) 243-7640
Fairfax Nursing Center 10701 Main St Fairfax, VA 22030 (703) 273-7705
Fountains at Washington House 5100 Fillmore Ave Alexandria, VA 22311 (703) 845-5000

Goodwin House Alexandria 4800 Fillmore Avenue Alexandria, VA 22311 (703) 824-1236
Goodwin House Bailey's Crossroads 3440 S. Jefferson Street Falls Church, VA 22041 (703) 578-7201
Heritage Hall Nursing & Rehab Center 122 Morven Park Rd NW Leesburg, VA 20176 (703) 777-8700
Iliff Nursing & Rehab Center 8000 Iliff Dr Dunn Loring, VA 22027 (703) 560-1000
INOVA Cameron Glen Care Center 1800 Cameron Glen Dr Reston, VA 20190 (703) 834-5800
INOVA Commonwealth Care Center 4315 Chain Bridge Rd Fairfax, VA 22030 (703) 934-5000
Jefferson, The 900 N Taylor St Arlington, VA 22203 (703) 516-9455

Leewood Healthcare Center 7120 Braddock Rd Annandale, VA 22003 (703) 256-9770
Loudoun Long Term Care Center 235 Old Waterford Rd NW Leesburg, VA 20176 (703) 771-2841
ManorCare Health Services - Alexandria 1510 Collingwood Rd Alexandria, VA 22308 (703) 765-6107
ManorCare Health Services - Arlington 550 S Carlin Springs Rd Arlington, VA 22204 (703) 379-7200
ManorCare Health Services - Fair Oaks 12475 Lee Jackson King Memorial Hwy Fairfax, VA 22033 (703) 352-7172
Mount Vernon Nursing Center 8111 Tiswell Dr Alexandria, VA 22306 (703) 360-4000
Potomac Center, Genesis ElderCare Network 1785 S Hayes St Arlington, VA 22202 (703) 920-5700

Ruxton Health of Alexandria 900 Virginia Ave Alexandria, VA 22302 (703) 684-9100
Ruxton Health of Woodbridge 14906 Jefferson Davis Hwy Woodbridge, VA 22191 (703) 491-6167
Sleepy Hollow Manor 6700 Columbia Pike Annandale, VA 22003 (703) 256-7000
Woodbine Rehabilitation & Healthcare Center 2729 King St Alexandria, VA 22302 (703) 836-8838

Central Virginia Nursing Homes

Amelia Nursing Home 8830 Virginia St Amelia, VA 23002 (804) 561-5611
Ashland Convalescent Center 906 Thompson St Ashland, VA 23005 (804) 798-3291

Avis B. Adams Christian Convalescent Center 200 Weaver Ave Emporia, VA 23847 (434) 634-6581
Battlefield Park Convalescent Center 250 Flank Rd Petersburg, VA 23805 (804) 861-2223
Beaufont Healthcare Center 200 Hioaks Rd Richmond, VA 23225 (804) 272-2918
Berry Hill Nursing Home 621 Berry Hill Rd South Boston, VA 24592 (434) 572-8901
Beth Sholom Home of Virginia 1600 John Rolfe Pkwy Richmond, VA 23233 (804) 750-2183
Brian Center Health & Rehab. - Lawrenceville 1722 Lawrenceville Plank Rd Lawrenceville, VA 23868 (434) 848-4766
Britthaven of Keysville 730 Lunenburg Hwy Keysville, VA 23947 (434) 736-8406

CLC Westhampton 1901 Libbie Ave Richmond, VA 23226 (804) 282-9767
Colonial Heights Health Care Center 831 Ellerslie Ave Colonial Heights, VA 23834 (804) 526-6851
Community Memorial Health Center 125 Buena Vista Circle South Hill, VA 23970 (434) 447-3151
Community Memorial Healthcenter /WS Hundley Annex 125 Buena Vista Circle South Hill, VA 23970 (434) 447-3151
Elizabeth Adam Crump Manor 3600 Mountain Rd Glen Allen, VA 23060 (804) 672-8725
Greensville Memorial Nursing Home 214 Weaver Ave Emporia, VA 23847 (434) 348-2000
Halifax Regional Hospital - Skilled Nursing Unit 2204 Willborn Ave South Boston, VA 24592 (434) 517-3100

Hanover Healthcare Center 8139 Lee Davis Rd Mechanicsville, VA 23111 (804) 559-5030
Health Care Center at Brandermill Woods 2100 Brandermill Pkwy Midlothian, VA 23112 (804) 379-7100
Health Care Center at Lucy Corr Village 6800 Lucy Corr Blvd Chesterfield, VA 23832 (804) 748-1511
Henrico HealthCare Center 561 N Airport Dr Highland Springs, VA 23075 (804) 737-0172
Heritage Hall - Blackstone 900 S Main St Blackstone, VA 23824 (434) 292-5301
Heritage Hall - Dillwyn 9 Brickyard Dr Dillwyn, VA 23936 (434) 983-2058
Holly Manor Nursing Home 2003 Cobb St Farmville, VA 23901 (434) 392-6106

Hopewell Health Care Center 905 Cousins Ave Hopewell, VA 23860 (804) 458-6325
John Randolph Nursing Home 409 W Randolph Rd Hopewell, VA 23860 (804) 452-3600
Laurels of Willow Creek 11611 Robious Rd Midlothian, VA 23113 (804) 379-4771
Lexington Court 1776 Cambridge Dr Richmond, VA 23233 (804) 740-6174
Little Sisters of the Poor/St Joseph' s Home 1503 Michael Rd Richmond, VA 23229 (804) 288-6245
ManorCare Health Services - Imperial 1719 Bellevue Ave Richmond, VA 23227 (804) 262-7364
ManorCare Health Services - Stratford Hall 2125 Hilliard Rd Richmond, VA 23228 (804) 266-9666

Meadows Nursing Center 2715 Dogtown Rd Goochland, VA 23063 (804) 556-4418
MeadowView Terrace 184 Buffalo Rd Clarksville, VA 23927 (434) 374-4141
Our Lady of Hope Health Center 13700 N Gayton Rd Richmond, VA 23233 (804) 360-1960
Parham Healthcare and Rehab. Center 2400 E Parham Rd Richmond, VA 23228 (804) 264-9185
Ruxton Health and Rehab. Center of Westover Hills 4403 Forest Hill Ave Richmond, VA 23225 (804) 231-0231
Ruxton of Stratford Hill 7246 Forest Hill Ave Richmond, VA 23225 (804) 320-7901
Seven Hills Health Care Center 1900 Cool Ln Richmond, VA 23223 (804) 343-6100

Southside Regional Medical Center - LTCU 801 S Adams St Petersburg, VA 23803 (804) 862-5000
Trinity Mission Health & Rehab of Farmville Route 5 Scott Dr Farmville, VA 23901 (434) 392-8806
Twin Oaks Convalescent Home 406 Oak Lane South Boston, VA 24592 (434) 572-2925
University Park 2420 Pemberton Rd Richmond, VA 23233 (804) 747-9200
Virginia Home, The 1101 Hampton St Richmond, VA 23220 (804) 359-4093
Walnut Hill Convalescent Center 287 S Boulevard Petersburg, VA 23805 (804) 733-1190
Waverly Healthcare Center 456 E Main St Waverly, VA 23890 (804) 834-3975

Westport Health Care Center 7300 Forest Ave Richmond, VA 23226 (804) 288-3152
Windsor, The 3600 Grove Ave Richmond, VA 23221 (804) 353-3881
Woodview, The 103 Rosehill Dr South Boston, VA 24592 (434) 572-4906

EASTERN VIRGINIA NURSING HOMES

Arcadia Nursing and Rehabilitation Center 17405 Lankford Hwy Nelsonia, VA 23414 (757) 665-5555
Autumn Care of Great Bridge 821 Cedar Rd Chesapeake, VA 23328 (757) 547-4528
Autumn Care of Norfolk 1401 Halstead Ave Norfolk, VA 23451 (757) 857-0481

Autumn Care of Portsmouth 3610 Winchester Dr Portsmouth, VA 23707 (757) 397-0725
Bay Pointe Medical and Rehab. Ctr. 1148 First Colonial Rd Virginia Beach, VA 23454 (757) 481-3321
Bayside Healthcare Center 1004 Independence Blvd Virginia Beach, VA 23455 (757) 464-4058
Bayside of Poquoson Convalescent Center 1 Vantage Dr Poquoson, VA 23662 (757) 868-9960
Beth Sholom Home of Eastern Virginia 6401 Auburn Dr Virginia Beach, VA 23464 (757) 420-2512
Beverly Manor of Portsmouth 900 London Boulevard Portsmouth, VA 23704 (757) 393-6864
Bon Secours DePaul Medical Ctr - Transitional Ctr 150 Kingsley Lane Norfolk, VA 23505 (757) 889-3200

Bon Secours-Maryview Nursing Care Center 4775 Bridge Rd Suffolk, VA 23435 (757) 215-1001
Chesapeake Healthcare Center 688 Kingsborough Square Chesapeake, VA 23320 (757) 547-9111
Chesapeake, The 955 Harpersville Rd Newport News, VA 23601 (757) 599-4376
CLC Tappahannock 1150 Marsh St Tappahannock, VA 22560 (804) 443-4308
Coliseum Park Nursing Home 305 Marcella Dr Hampton, VA 23666 (757) 827-8953
Courtland Healthcare Center 23020 S Main St Courtland, VA 23837 (757) 653-0908
Harbour Pointe Medical and Rehab. Ctr. 1005 Hampton Blvd Norfolk, VA 23507 (757) 623-5602

Heritage Hall - Nassawadox 9468 Hospital Rd Nassawadox, VA 23413 (757) 442-5600
Heritage Hall - Virginia Beach 5580 Daniel Smith Rd Virginia Beach, VA 23462 (757) 499-7029
James River Convalescent Center 540 Aberthaw Ave Newport News, VA 23601 (757) 595-2273
Lake Taylor Transitional Care Hospital 1309 Kempsville Rd Norfolk, VA 23502 (757) 461-5001
Lancashire Convalescent & Rehab Center 287 School St Kilmarnock, VA 22482 (804) 435-1684
Mary Washington Senior Living Community 2400 McKinney Blvd Colonial Beach, VA 22443 (804) 224-2222
Mizpah Nursing Home 74 Mizpah Road Locust Hill, VA 23092 (804) 758-5260

Nansemond Pointe Rehab. & Healthcare Ctr. 200 W Constance Rd Suffolk, VA 23434 (757) 539-8744
Newport News Nursing & Rehab Center 12997 Nettles Dr Newport News, VA 23602 (757) 249-8880
Newport, The 11141 Warwick Boulevard Newport News, VA 23601 (757) 595-3733
Norfolk Healthcare Center 901 E Princess Anne Rd Norfolk, VA 23504 (757) 626-1642
Northampton Convalescent Center 1028 Topping Lane Hampton, VA 23666 (757) 826-4922
Oakwood Nursing and Rehab Center 5520 Indian River Rd Virginia Beach, VA 23464 (757) 420-3600
Orchard, The 20 Delfae Dr Warsaw, VA 22572 (804) 313-2500

Our Lady of Perpetual Help Health Center 4560 Princess Anne Rd Virginia Beach, VA 23462 (757) 495-4211
Regency Healthcare Center 112 N Constitution Dr Yorktown, VA 23692 (757) 890-0675
River Pointe Rehab. and Healthcare Ctr. 4142 Bonney Rd Virginia Beach, VA 23452 (757) 340-0620
Riverside Convalescent Center - Hampton 414 Algonquin Rd Hampton, VA 23661 (757) 722-9881
Riverside Convalescent Center - Mathews Route 611 and 14 Mathews, VA 23109 (804) 725-9443
Riverside Convalescent Center - Saluda 672 Gloucester Road Saluda, VA 23149 (804) 758-2363
Riverside Convalescent Center - Smithfield 200 Lumar Rd Smithfield, VA 23430 (757) 357-3282

Riverside Convalescent Center - West Point 2960 Chelsea Rd West Point, VA 23181 (804) 843-4323
Riverside Regional Convalescent Center 1000 Old Denbigh Blvd Newport News, VA 23602 (757) 875-2000
Riverside Tappahannock Hospital - LTCU Tappahannock, VA 22560 (804) 443-3311
Seaside, The Health Center at Atlantic Shores 1200 Atlantic Shores Dr Virginia Beach, VA 23454 (757) 716-2060
Sentara Nursing Center - Chesapeake 776 Oak Grove Rd Chesapeake, VA 23320 (757) 204-4000
Sentara Nursing Center - Hampton 2230 Executive Dr Hampton, VA 23666 (757) 224-2230
Sentara Nursing Center - Norfolk 249 S Newtown Rd Norfolk, VA 23502 (757) 892-5500

Sentara Nursing Center - Portsmouth 4201 Greenwood Dr Portsmouth, VA 23701 (757) 673-5000
Sentara Nursing Center - Virginia Beach 3750 Sentara Way Virginia Beach, VA 23452 (757) 306-2700
Sentara Nursing Center - Windermere 1604 Old Donation Pkwy Virginia Beach, VA 23454 (757) 496-3939
Shore Lifecare at Parksley 26181 Parksley Rd Parksley, VA 23421 (757) 665-5133
Shore Memorial Hospital - LTCU 9507 Hospital Ave Nassawadox, VA 23413 (757) 442-8000
Southampton Memorial Hospital - LTCU 100 Fairview Dr Franklin, VA 23851 (757) 596-6100
St. Francis Nursing Center 4 Ridgewood Pkwy Newport News, VA 23602 (757) 886-6500

St. Mary's Home for Disabled Children 317 Chapel St Norfolk, VA 23504 (757) 622-2208
Stanleytown Healthcare Center 240 Riverside Dr Stanleytown, VA 23504 (276) 629-1772
SunBridge Care & Rehab for Chesapeake 1017 N George Washington Hwy Chesapeake, VA 23323 (757) 485-5500
Tandem Health Care at Williamsburg 1811 Jamestown Rd Williamsburg, VA 23185 (757) 229-9991
Tandem Health Care of Norfolk 3900 Llewellyn Ave Norfolk, VA 23504 (757) 625-5363
Tandem Health Care of Windsor 23352 Courthouse Hwy Windsor, VA 23487 (757) 242-4770
Thornton Hall 827 Norview Ave Norfolk, VA 23509 (757) 853-6281

Virginia Beach Healthcare & Rehab Center 1801 Camelot Dr Virginia Beach, VA 23454 (757) 481-3500
Virginia Shores Health Care & Rehab 340 Lynn Shores Dr Virginia Beach, VA 23452 (757) 340-6611
Walter Reed Convalescent Center 7602 Meredith Dr Gloucester, VA 23061 (804) 693-6503
Warsaw Healthcare Center 5373 Richmond Rd Warsaw, VA 22572 (804) 333-3616
Williamsburg Center 1235 Mount Vernon Ave Williamsburg, VA 23185 (757) 229-4121
York Convalescent Center 113 Battle Rd Yorktown, VA 23692 (757) 898-1491

NORTHWESTERN VIRGINIA NURSING HOMES

Augusta Medical Center - Skilled Nursing Unit 96 Medical Care Dr Fishersville, VA 22939 (540) 932-4000
Augusta Nursing & Rehab Center 83 Crossroads Ln Fishersville, VA 22939 (540) 885-8434
Autumn Care of Madison 1 Autumn Court Madison, VA 22727 (540) 948-3054
Avanté at Harrisonburg 94 South Ave Harrisonburg, VA 22801 (540) 433-2791
Avanté of Waynesboro 1221 Rosser Ave Waynesboro, VA 22980 (540) 949-7191
Beverly HealthCare Fredericksburg 3900 Plank Rd Fredericksburg, VA 22407 (540) 786-8351
Bowling Green Health Care Center 120 Anderson Ave Bowling Green, VA 22427 (804) 633-4839

Brooke Nursing Center 140 Andrew Chapell Rd Stafford, VA 22554 (540) 657-0019
Cedars Nursing Home, The 1242 Cedars Ct Charlottesville, VA 22901 (434) 296-5611
Culpeper Health & Rehab Center 602 Madison Rd Culpeper, VA 22701 (540) 825-2884
Evergreen Health and Rehab. of Winchester 380 Millwood Ave Winchester, VA 22601 (540) 667-7010
Evergreene Nursing Care Center 355 William Mills Dr Stanardsville, VA 22973 (434) 985-4434
Harrisonburg Health & Rehab Center 1225 S Reservoir St Harrisonburg, VA 22801 (540) 433-2623
Heritage Hall - Charlottesville 505 W Rio Rd Charlottesville, VA 22901 (434) 978-7015

Heritage Hall - Front Royal 400 W Strasburg Rd Front Royal, VA 22630 (540) 636-3700
Heritage Hall - King George 8443 King's Hwy King George, VA 22485 (540) 775-4000
Heritage Hall - Lexington 205 Houston St Lexington, VA 24450 (540) 464-8181
Hillcrest Manor Nursing Home 110 Lauck Dr Winchester, VA 22603 (540) 667-7830
King's Daughter Community Health & Rehab Center 1410 N Augusta St Staunton, VA 24401 (540) 886-6233
Life Care Center of New Market 315 E Lee Hwy New Market, VA 22844 (540) 740-8041
Louisa Healthcare Center 210 Elm St Louisa, VA 23093 (540) 967-2250

Lovingston Healthcare Center 393 Front St Lovingston, VA 22949 (434) 263-4823
Martha Jefferson House 1600 Gordon Ave Charlottesville, VA 22903 (434) 293-6136
MontVue Nursing Home 30 Montvue Dr Luray, VA 22835 (540) 743-4571
Mountain View Nursing Home Route 607, Elly Road Aroda, VA 22709 (540) 948-6831
Oak Hill Center 512 Houston St Staunton, VA 24401 (540) 886-2335
Oak Lea Nursing Home 1475 Virginia Ave Harrisonburg, VA 22802 (540) 564-3500
Oak Springs of Warrenton 614 Hastings Ln Warrenton, VA 20186 (540) 347-4770

Orange County Nursing Home and Home for Adults 120 Dogwood Ln Orange, VA 22960 (540) 672-2611
Our Lady of Peace 751 Hillsdale Dr Charlottesville, VA 22901 (434) 973-1155
Rose Hill Nursing Center 110 Chalmers Ct Berryville, VA 22611 (540) 955-9995
Shenandoah Nursing Home 339 Westminister Dr Fishersville, VA 22939 (540) 949-8665
Shenandoah, Valley Health Care Center 3737 Catalpa Ave Buena Vista, VA 24416 (540) 261-7444
Skyline Terrace Convalescent Home 123 Lakeview Rd Woodstock, VA 22664 (540) 459-3738
Springs Nursing Center Spring St Hot Springs, VA 24445 (540) 839-2299

Tandem Health Care of Woodstock 803 S Main St Woodstock, VA 22664 (540) 459-5676
Trinity Mission Health & Rehab of Charlottesville 1150 Northwest Dr Charlottesville, VA 22901 (434) 973-7933
Village Nursing Center Rt 15 Fork Union, VA 23055 (434) 842-2916
Warren Memorial Hospital - Lynn Care Ctr 1000 Shenandoah Ave Front Royal, VA 22630 (540) 636-0300
Warrenton Overlook Health and Rehab Center 360 Hospital Dr Warrenton, VA 20186 (540) 349-1919
Woodmont Center 11 Dairy Ln Fredericksburg, VA 22405 (540) 371-9414

Southwestern Virginia Nursing Homes

Appomattox Healthcare Center 215 Evergreen Ave Appomattox, VA 24522 (434) 352-7420
Asbury Place 990 Holston Rd Wytheville, VA 24382 (276) 228-5595
Autumn Care of Altavista 1317 Lola Ave Altavista, VA 24517 (434) 369-6651
Avanté at Lynchburg 2081 Langhorne Rd Lynchburg, VA 24501 (434) 846-8437
Avanté at Roanoke 324 King George Ave SW Roanoke, VA 24016 (540) 345-8139
Bedford County Nursing Home 1229 County Farm Rd Bedford, VA 24523 (540) 586-7658
Berkshire Healthcare Center 705 Clearview Dr Vinton, VA 24179 (540) 982-6691

Beverly Health Care - Blue Ridge 836 Glendale Rd Galax, VA 24333 (276) 236-9991
Beverly HealthCare - Martinsville 1607 Spruce St Martinsville, VA 24112 (276) 632-7146
Beverly HealthCare - Ridgecrest Ross Carter Blvd Duffield, VA 24244 (276) 431-2841
Blue Ridge Nursing Center 105 Landmark Drive Stuart, VA 24171 (276) 694-7161
Blue Ridge Rehab Center 300 Blue Ridge St Martinsville, VA 24112 (276) 638-8701
Brian Center Health & Rehab - Alleghany 100 Alleghany Regional Hospital Lan Low Moor, VA 24457 (540) 862-3610
Brian Center Health & Rehab - Scott County 105 Clonce St Weber City, VA 24290 (276) 386-9444

Brian Center Nursing Care - Fincastle 188 Old Fincastle Rd Fincastle, VA 24090 (540) 473-2288
Carilion Giles Memorial Hospital 1 Taylor Avenue Pearisburg, VA 24134 (540) 921-6000
Carrington, The 2406 Atherholt Rd Lynchburg, VA 24501 (434) 846-3200
Clinch, Valley Medical Center - LTCU 2949 W Front St Richlands, VA 24641 (276) 596-6000
Duffield Adult Residential & Nursing Facility Ross Carter Blvd Duffield, VA 24244 (276) 431-4200
Edgemont Center 100 Edgemont Rd Wytheville, VA 24382 (276) 228-7380
Fairmont Crossing Rehab & Healthcare Center 173 Brockman Park Dr Amherst, VA 24521 (434) 946-2850

Francis Marion Manor 100 Francis Marion Ln Marion, VA 24354 (276) 782-1395
Franklin Healthcare Center 720 Orchard Ave Rocky Mount, VA 24151 (540) 489-3467
Grace Healthcare of Abingdon 600 Walden Rd Abingdon, VA 24210 (276) 628-2111
Grace Lodge 1503 Grace St Lynchburg, VA 24505 (434) 528-0969
Grayson Nursing & Rehabilitation Center 400 S Independence Ave Independence, VA 24348 (276) 773-0303
Gretna Healthcare Center 595 Vaden Dr Gretna, VA 24557 (434) 656-1206
Guggenheimer Nursing Home 1902 Grace St Lynchburg, VA 24504 (434) 947-5100

Heritage Hall - Big Stone Gap 2045 Valley View Dr Big Stone Gap, VA 24219 (276) 523-3000
Heritage Hall - Blacksburg 3610 S Main St Blacksburg, VA 24060 (540) 951-7000
Heritage Hall - Brookneal 633 Cook Ave Brookneal, VA 24528 (434) 376-3717
Heritage Hall - Clintwood Route 607 Clintwood, VA 24228 (276) 926-4693
Heritage Hall - Grundy Route 5, Box 104 Grundy, VA 24614 (276) 935-8144
Heritage Hall - Laurel Meadows 16600 Danville Pike Laurel Fork, VA 24352 (276) 398-2117
Heritage Hall - Tazewell 121 Ben Bolt Ave Tazewell, VA 24651 (276) 988-2515

Heritage Hall - Wise 9434 Coeburn Mountain Rd Wise, VA 24293 (276) 328-2721
Highland Ridge Rehab Center 5872 Hanks Ave Dublin, VA 24084 (540) 674-4193
Kegley Manor Route 1 Bastian, VA 24314 (276) 688-4141
Kroontje Health Care Center, The 1000 Litton Ln Blacksburg, VA 24060 (540) 953-3200
Lee Nursing & Rehab Center 1751 Combs Rd Pennington Gap, VA 24277 (276) 546-4566
Liberty House Nursing Home - Clifton Forge 1725 Main St Clifton Forge, VA 24422 (540) 862-5791
Lynchburg Health & Rehab Center 5615 Seminole Ave Lynchburg, VA 24502 (434) 239-2657

Maple Grove Health Care Center 230 SE Main St Lebanon, VA 24266 (276) 889-0733
Medical Care Center 2200 Landover Place Lynchburg, VA 24501 (434) 846-4626
NHC Healthcare, Bristol 245 North St Bristol, VA 24201 (276) 669-4711
Oakwood Manor - LTCU 1613 Oakwood St Bedford, VA 24523 (540) 586-2441
Our Lady of the Valley 650 N Jefferson St Roanoke, VA 24016 (540) 345-5111
Pheasant Ridge Nursing Home 4355 Pheasant Ridge Rd SW Roanoke, VA 24014 (540) 725-8210
Piney Forest Healthcare Center 450 Piney Forest Rd Danville, VA 24540 (434) 799-1565

Pulaski Community Hospital 2400 Lee Hwy Pulaski, VA 24301 (540) 980-6822
Pulaski Health & Rehabilitation Center 2401 Lee Hwy Pulaski, VA 24301 (540) 980-3111
Radford Nursing and Rehab Center 700 Randolph St Radford, VA 24141 (540) 633-6533
Raleigh Court Healthcare Center 1527 Grandin Rd SW Roanoke, VA 24015 (540) 342-9525
Richfield Recovery and Care Center 3615 W Main St Salem, VA 24153 (540) 380-4500
Riverside Health and Rehab Center 2344 Riverside Dr Danville, VA 24540 (434) 791-3800
Riverview Nursing Home 120 Virginia Ave Rich Creek, VA 24147 (540) 726-2328

RJ Reynolds - Patrick Co Mem Hospital - LTCU 18688 Jeb Stuart Hwy Stuart, VA 24171 (276) 694-8678
Roman Eagle Memorial Home 2526 N Main St Danville, VA 24540 (434) 836-9510
Salem Health & Rehabilitation Center 1945 Roanoke Blvd Salem, VA 24153 (540) 345-3894
Skyline Manor Nursing Home 237 Franklin Pike Rd SE Floyd, VA 24091 (540) 745-2016
Smyth Co Comm. Hospital - LTCU 565 Radio Hill Rd Marion, VA 24354 (276) 782-1234
Snyder Nursing Home 11 N Broad St Salem, VA 24153 (540) 389-0160
South Roanoke Nursing Home 3823 Franklin Rd SW Roanoke, VA 24014 (540) 344-4325

St. John's Nursing Home 3500 Powhatan St Lynchburg, VA 24501 (434) 845-6045
St. Mary's Hospital Norton - LTCU Third St, NE Norton, VA 24273 (276) 679-9100
Trinity Mission Health & Rehab of Hillsville 222 Fulcher St Hillsville, VA 24343 (276) 728-2486
Trinity Mission Health & Rehab of Rocky Mount 300 Hatcher St Rocky Mount, VA 24151 (540) 483-9261
Valley Health Care Center 940 E Lee Hwy Chilhowie, VA 24319 (276) 646-8911
Virginia Baptist Hospital - LTCU 3300 Rivermont Ave Lynchburg, VA 24503 (434) 947-4000
Virginia Veterans Care Center 4550 Shenandoah Ave NW Roanoke, VA 24017 (540) 982-2860

Waddell Nursing Home 202 Painter St Galax, VA 24333 (276) 236-5164
Westwood Center Westwood Medical Park Bluefield, VA 24605 (276) 322-5439
Woodhaven Nursing Home 13055 W Lynchburg/Salem Tpke Montvale, VA 24122 (540) 947-2207
Woodlands, The 1000 Fairview Heights Clifton Forge, VA 24422 (540) 863-4096
Wythe Co Community Hospital - LTCU 600 W Ridge Rd Wytheville, VA 24382 (276) 228-0200

APPENDIX B — VIRGINIA & NATIONAL RESOURCES

AARP 601 E St., NW Washington, D.C. 20049 Telephone: 202-434-2277 www.aarp.org *A national membership organization whose purpose is to enhance the quality of life for persons over age 50, promote independence, and improve the image of aging.*
Alzheimer's Association National Capitol Area 11240 Waples Mill Road, Suite 402 Fairfax, Virginia 22030 Telephone: 703-359-4440 Toll-free: 866-259-0042 www.alz-nca.org *The Alzheimer's Association is the premier source of information and support for Americans with Alzheimer's disease and related disorders.*
Eldercare Locator Toll Free: 800-677-1116 www.eldercare.gov *A public service of the U.S. Administration on Aging designed to help identify community resources for seniors and their caregivers anywhere in the U.S.*

Guide to Retirement Living
Douglas Publishing Company
P.O. Box 7512
McLean, VA 22106-7512
Tel: 800-394-9990
www.retirement-living.com
A publication listing senior housing, home care, and other resources for older persons in the metropolitan Washington, D.C. area. Free copies are available at Senior Centers, Churches, or by contacting the publisher.

Hispanic Committee of Virginia
5827 Columbia Pike, Suite 200
Falls Church, VA 22041
Telephone: 703-671-5666
www.hispaniccommitteeofvirginia.org
Offers information and referral services, interpreters, and varied assistance to Spanish-speaking persons.

Medicare
Toll Free: 800-633-4227
TTY: 877-486-2048
www.medicare.gov
Medicare has two parts:
Part A is hospital insurance, which helps to pay hospital bills and some follow-up care.
Part B is medical insurance, which helps to pay doctors' bills and other services.

Medicare Nursing Home Compare Web Site
Online nursing home comparison tool.
www.medicare.gov/NHCompare

Mid-Atlantic Geriatric Care Managers Association Telephone: 520-881-8008 www.gcmonline.org *A group of professionals trained in the field of human services who are dedicated to promoting the advancement of dignified care for older adults. Members are certified or licensed at the independent practice level. Serve older adults and their families on a fee-for-service basis throughout Maryland, Virginia, and Washington, DC.*
National Citizens' Coalition for Nursing Home Reform 1424 16th Street, NW Washington, D.C. 20036-2211 Telephone: 202-332-2275 *A non-profit group whose mission is to improve the quality of care and quality of life for residents in nursing homes. Will provide consumer information upon request.*
Northern Virginia Information Line of the Jewish Council for the Aging Telephone: 703-425-0999 *Assists older adults and their families by referring them to services and programs.*
Northern Virginia Long-Term Care Ombudsman 12011 Gov't Center Pkwy, Suite 708 Fairfax, VA 22035 Telephone: 703-324-5861 TTY: 800-828-1140 *Inspects health care facilities, programs and services for compliance with federal and state regulations; investigates consumer complaints regarding quality of health care services.*

Personal Advocate Service
A program sponsored by the Arlington Agency on Aging to assist Arlington residents 60 and over and their families to identify and access community services by using trained volunteers. Includes volunteers specially trained about Medicare, Medigap, Managed Care, and Long-Term Care Insurance.
Telephone: 703-228-1700
TTY: 703-228-1788

Social Security Administration
Toll Free: 800-772-1213
TTY: 800-325-0778
www.ssa.gov
May pay cash benefits to people who are unable to work for a year or more because of a disability.

Virginia State Bureau of Insurance
Toll Free: 800-552-7945
For questions about Medicare supplementary insurance and long-term care insurance policies, as well as complaints about alleged insurance abuses.

Virginia Board of Nursing Home Administrators
Telephone: 804-662-7457
TTY: 804-662-7197
Complaints: 800-533-1560
Licensing body for nursing home administrators in Virginia; accepts complaints.

Virginia Department of Medical Assistance Services
600 East Broad Street
Richmond, VA 23219
Telephone: 804-786-4231
http://165.176.249.159

Virginia Department of Social Services *Agency responsible for taking Medicaid applications.* Telephone: 800-230-6977 www.dss.state.va.us/benefit/medicaid.html
Virginia Health Information www.vhi.org *Listing of all Nursing Homes in Virginia with link to Medicare's Nursing Home Compare Web site.*

APPENDIX C — AREA AGENCIES ON AGING

Alexandria Agency on Aging 2525 Mount Vernon Avenue Alexandria, VA 22301 Telephone: 703-838-0920 http://ci.alexandria.va.us/dhs/community_partners/aging_netwk.html **Local Area Served:** City of Alexandria
Appalachian Agency for Senior Citizens 216 College Ridge Road P.O. Box 765 Cedar Bluff, VA 24609-0765 Telephone: 276-964-4915 TTY: 276-964-5765 Toll-Free: 800-656-2272 www.aasc.org **Local Areas Served:** Counties of Buchanan, Dickenson, Russell and Tazewell
Arlington Agency on Aging 3033 Wilson Boulevard Suite 700-B Arlington, VA 22201 Telephone: 703-228-1700 www.co.arlington.va.us/dhs **Local Area Served**: County of Arlington

Bay Aging 5306 Old Virginia Street P.O. Box 610 Urbanna, VA 23175-0610 Telephone: 804-758-2386 www.bayaging.org **Local Areas Served:** Counties of Essex, Gloucester, King and Queen, King William, Lancaster, Mathews, Middlesex, Northumberland, Richmond and Westmoreland.
Central Virginia Area Agency on Aging 3024 Forest Hills Circle Lynchburg, VA 24501-2312 Telephone: 434-385-9070 www.cvaaa.com **Local Areas Served**: Counties of Amherst, Appomattox, Bedford and Campbell. Cities of Bedford and Lynchburg
Crater District Area Agency on Aging 23 Seyler Drive Petersburg, VA 23805-9243 Telephone: 804-732-7020 www.cdaaa.org **Local Areas Served**: Counties of Dinwiddie, Greensville, Prince George, Surry and Sussex. Cities of Colonial Heights, Emporia, Hopewell and Petersburg.
District Three Senior Services 4453 Lee Highway Marion, VA 24354-4269 Telephone: 276-783-8157 Toll-Free: 800-541-0933 www.district-three.org **Local Areas Served**: Counties of Bland, Carroll, Grayson, Smyth, Washington and Wythe. Cities of Bristol and Galax.

Eastern Shore Agency on Aging 36282 Lankford Highway, Suite 13-D P.O. Box 415 Belle Haven, VA 23306-0415 Telephone: 757-442-9652 Toll-Free: 800-452-5977 **Local Areas Served:** Counties of Accomack and Northampton.
Fairfax Area Agency on Aging Human Services Building, B-3, 7th Floor 12011 Government Center Parkway Fairfax, VA 22035 www.fairfaxcounty.gov/service/aaa Tel: 703-324-5411 **Toll-Free:** 866-503-0217 **Local Areas Served**: County of Fairfax, Cities of Fairfax and Falls Church
Jefferson Area Board For Aging 674 Hillsdale Drive, Suite 9 Charlottesville, VA 22901-1799 Telephone: 434-817-5222 www.jabacares.org **Local Areas Served:** Counties of Albemarle, Fluvanna, Greene, Louisa, and Nelson; City of Charlottesville.
Lake Country Area Agency on Aging 1105 West Danville Street South Hill, VA 23970-3501 434-447-7661 Toll-Free: 800-252-4464 www.lcaaa.org **Local Areas Served**: Counties of Brunswick, Halifax and Mecklenburg.

LOA Area Agency on Aging
706 Campbell Avenue, SW
P.O. Box 14205
Roanoke, VA 24038-4205
Telephone: 540-345-0451
www.loaa.org
Local Areas Served: Counties of Alleghany, Botetourt, Craig, and Roanoke. Cities of Covington, Roanoke and Salem.

Loudoun County Area Agency on Aging
102 Heritage Way, NE, Suite 102
Leesburg, VA 20176
Telephone: 703-777-0257
www.co.loudoun.va.us/prcs/aaa/index.htm
Local Areas Served: County of Loudoun

Mountain Empire Older Citizens
Block 1-A Industrial Park Road
P.O. Box 888
Big Stone Gap, VA 24219-0888
Telephone: 276-523-4202
Toll-Free: 800-252-6362
www.meoc.org
Local Areas Served: Counties of Lee, Scott and Wise. City of Norton.

New River Valley Agency on Aging
141 East Main Street
Pulaski, VA 24301-5029
Telephone: 540-980-7720
Toll-Free: 866-260-4417
Local Areas Served: Counties of Floyd, Giles, Montgomery and Pulaski. City of Radford.

Peninsula Agency on Aging
739 Thimble Shoals Boulevard
Executive Center Bldg 1000, Suite 1006
Newport News, VA 23606-3585
Telephone: 757-873-0541
www.paainc.org
Local Areas Served: Counties of James City and York. Cities of Hampton, Newport News, Poquoson and Williamsburg.

Piedmont Senior Resources Area Agency on Aging
Inverness Road & Route 624
P.O. Box 398
Burkeville, VA 23922-0398
Telephone: 434-767-5588
Toll-Free: 800-995-6918
Local Areas Served: Counties of Amelia, Buckingham, Charlotte, Cumberland, Lunenburg, Nottoway, and Prince Edward.

Prince William Area Agency on Aging
7987 Ashton Avenue, Suite 204
Manassas, VA 22110
Local Areas Served: County of Prince William. Cities of Manassas and Manassas Park.
Telephone: 703-792-6400
www.pwcgov.org/aoa

Rappahannock-Rapidan Area Agency on Aging 15361 Bradford Road P.O. Box 1568 Culpeper, VA 22701-1568 Telephone: 540-825-3100 TDD: 540-825-7391 **Local Areas Served:** Counties of Culpeper, Fauquier, Madison, Orange and Rappahannock.
Rappahannock Area Agency on Aging 171 Warrenton Road Fredericksburg, VA 22405-1343 Telephone: 540-371-3375 Toll-Free: 800-262-4012 raaa.home.infionline.net **Local Areas Served:** Counties of Caroline, King George, Spotsylvania and Stafford. City of Fredericksburg.
Senior Services of Southeastern Virginia Interstate Corporate Center, Bldg. 5 6350 Center Drive, Suite 101 Norfolk, VA 23502-4101 Telephone: 757-461-9481 www.ssseva.org **Local Areas Served:** Counties of Isle of Wight and Southampton. Cities of Chesapeake, Franklin, Norfolk, Portsmouth, Suffolk, and Virginia Beach.

Shenandoah Area Agency on Aging 207 Mosby Lane Front Royal, VA 22630-3029 Telephone: 540-635-7141 Toll-Free: 800-883-4122 www.shenandoahaaa.com **Local Areas Served:** Counties of Clarke, Frederick, Page, Shenandoah and Warren. City of Winchester.
Southern Area Agency on Aging 433 Commonwealth Boulevard E, Suite A Martinsville, VA 24112-2020 Telephone: 276-632-6442 Toll-Free: 800-468-4571 www.southernaaa.org **Local Areas Served:** Counties of Franklin, Henry, Patrick and Pittsylvania. Cities of Danville and Martinsville.
The Capital Area Agency on Aging 24 East Cary Street Richmond, VA 23219-3796 Telephone: 804-343-3000 Toll-Free: 800-989-2286 www.seniorconnections-va.org **Local Areas Served:** Counties of Charles City, Chesterfield, Goochland, Hanover, Henrico, New Kent and Powhatan. City of Richmond.

Valley Program for Aging Services 325 Pine Avenue P.O. Box 817 Waynesboro, VA 22980-0603 Telephone: 540-949-7141 Toll-Free: 800-868-8727 **Local Areas Served:** Counties of Augusta, Bath, Highland, Rockbridge and Rockingham. Cities of Buena Vista, Harrisonburg, Lexington, Staunton and Waynesboro.
Virginia Department for the Aging Telephone: 800-552-3402 TTY: 804-662-9333 www.vda.virginia.gov *State agency that administers federal Older Americans Act funds and related state funding distributed to area agencies on aging and other organizations.*
Virginia Association of Area Agencies on Aging 530 E. Main Street Richmond, VA 23219 Telephone: 804-644-2804 *The state association for the 25 Area Agencies in Virginia. Manages the state Long-Term Care Ombudsman Program, which assists in resolving problems in long term care facilities.*

APPENDIX D — ELDER ABUSE RESOURCES

Virginia Elder Abuse Hotline 888-83-ADULT (888-832-3858) Out-of-state: 804-371-0896 Run by Virginia Department of Social Services Adult Protective Services Program. Operates 24-hours per day, 7 days per week, 365 days per year.
Virginia TRIAD (804) 786-3344 (voice) www.oag.state.va.us/Protecting/Triad/contacts2.htm This local and regional coalition, linked to a statewide and national TRIAD movement to prevent crime against elderly persons, represents a partnership among AARP, International Association of Chiefs of Police, and the National Sheriffs' Association. A major purpose of TRIAD is to develop, expand and implement effective crime prevention and education programs for older Virginians.
National Center on Elder Abuse www.elderabusecenter.org 202-898-2586
TLC 4 Long Term Care www.tlc4ltc.org 703-569-1746
Virginia Friends & Relatives of NH Residents 804-644-2804
Citizens Committee to Protect the Elderly www.citizenscommittee.org 757-518-8500

Appendix E — Geriatricians

Dr. Linda Abbey (Midlothian)
Dr. Cheryl Arenella (Centreville)
Dr. Dwight Bailey (Lebanon)
Dr. James Barton (Williamsburg)
Dr. James Bell (Pennington Gap)
Dr. Alexander Berger (Portsmouth)
Dr. Richard Bikowski (Portsmouth)
Dr. Maurice Blackburn (Mechanicsville)
Dr. Daniel Bluestein (Norfolk)
Dr. Soheir Boshra (Roanoke)
Dr. Deborah Bostock (Yorktown)
Dr. Floyd Bradd (Front Royal)
Dr. Stanley Brittman (Norfolk)
Dr. Jai Cho (Ivy)
Dr. Joanne Crantz (Fairfax)
Dr. Louis Croteau (Virginia Beach)
Dr. James Dixon (Norfolk)
Dr. Damien Doyle (Annandale)
Dr. Charles Driscoll (Lynchburg)

Dr. Mohamad El-Masri (Richmond)
Dr. Myron Eller (Martinsville)
Dr. Kurtis Elward (Charlottesville)
Dr. Gregory Estlund (Portsmouth)
Dr. Hugo Falcon (Geriatric Psychiatry - Burkeville)
Dr. Howard Feldman (Virginia Beach)
Dr. Page Fletcher (Geriatric Psychiatry - Purcellville)
Dr. James Forrester (Callao)
Dr. Stanley Furman (Richmond)
Dr. Sim Galazka (Charlottesville)
Dr. John Gazewood (Charlottesville)
Dr. Monica Gilbert (Roanoke)
Dr. Louis Graham (Lynchburg)
Dr. Thomas Grant (Norfolk)
Dr. John Hagy (Rocky Mount)
Dr. Christopher Heck (Waynesboro)
Dr. Laura Heiby (Virginia Beach)
Dr. David Hoshino (Oak Hall)
Dr. William Jackson (Suffolk)
Dr. Frank Johnson (Bluefield)
Dr. Barbara Kalazny (Falls Church)

Dr. Howard Kimes (Dunn Loring)
Dr. John Kugler (Fredericksburg)
Dr. Deborah Leavens (Herndon)
Dr. David Leonard (Fairfax)
Dr. Joanne Lynn (Arlington)
Dr. Gagan Mall (Geriatric Psychiatry - Midlothian)
Dr. Olivia Mansilla (Richmond)
Dr. Terence McCormally (Fairfax)
Dr. Jennifer Nau (Gainesville)
Dr. Hien Nguyen (Fairfax)
Dr. Gerald Nowak, DO (Alexandria)
Dr. Sharon Petitjean (Newport News)
Dr. Hiep Pham (Roanoke)
Dr. Patricia Pletke (Lynchburg)
Dr. William Plonk (Waynesboro)
Dr. John Pope (Richmond)
Dr. Cissy Pottanat (Falls Church)
Dr. Muhammad Raja (Midlothian)
Dr. Swarna Reddy (Geriatric Psychiatry - Herndon)
Dr. James Redington (Hot Springs)
Dr. Charles Rosenfarb (Dulles)

Dr. Walid Saado (Clintwood)
Dr. Richard Sokol (Norfolk)
Dr. Michael Sotosky (Chesapeake)
Dr. Holly Stanley (Richmond)
Dr. Anthony Stavola (Roanoke)
Dr. Angela Stiltner (Gordonsville)
Dr. Girard Thompson (Chatham)
Dr. Clara Toothman (Bristol)
Dr. Brian Unwin (Fairfax)
Dr. Lawrence Varner (Farmville)
Dr. Kenneth Walker (Pearisburg)
Dr. Roger Westfall (Front Royal)
Dr. Gary Williams (Norton)
Dr. Stephen Willing (Crozet)
Dr. Samuel Wittenberg (Virginia Beach)

APPENDIX F — GERIATRIC CARE MANAGERS

Barbara Adams / Choices for Aging Falls Church / 703-241-4100 www.choicesforaging.com
Kathleen Allen / Senior Care Management Services, LLC Alexandria / 703-329-0900 www.seniorcarems.com
A. Alston / Family Management Services, Inc. Fairfax / 703-352-3013 www.familymgmt.com
Linda Aufderhaar / Senior Care Associates Fairfax / 703-502-0240 www.seniorcare-associates.com
Donna Barrette / Generation Solutions Lynchburg / 434-455-6500
Judith Burkitt / GeriatriCare Management, Inc. Arlington / 703-538-5342 www.geriatricare.com
Kate Caldwell / ElderTree, LLC Sterling / 703-220-8846 www.eldertreecare.com
Shannon Campanelli / Ann O'Neil & Associates Falls Church / 703-237-9048
Marva Davis / Adult Companion Care Alexandria / 703-549-7894

Gale Davis / Senior Connections Richmond / 804-343-3056 www.seniorconnections-va.org
Barbie DeVellis / Generation Solutions Roanoke / 540-776-3622
Margaret Duffy Virginia Beach / 757-460-5885
Laurie Duncan / Choices for Aging Falls Church / 703-241-4100 www.choicesforaging.com
Marilyn Fall / Elder Care at Home, Inc. Virginia Beach / 757-464-4800 www.geriatriccaremanagement.net
Marsha Grant / Cleansing Water, Inc. Warrenton / 540-341-0212
Marjorie Harper / ElderLink Options for Caregiving Fairfax / 703-324-5376
Helen Hipps Reston / 703-502-0240
Janet Horgen / Home Management Services, Inc. Arlington / 703-838-0038
Rhoda Hurst / By Your Side Home Health, Inc Blacksburg / 540-765-7369
Jane Kallio / Jewish Family Services Richmond / 804-282-5644
Norah Knutsen / Mature Options, Inc. Glen Allen / 804-282-0753

Clare Krell / Jewish Family Service of Tidewater Norfolk / 757-489-3111
Joan Mitchell / Care Management for the Elderly Yorktown / 757-865-7159
Louise Mohardt / Geriatric Support Services Lancaster / 804-462-7730 www.geriatricsupportservices.com
Constance O'Connor / GeriatriCare Management, Inc. Arlington / 703-524-0752 www.geriatricare.com
Ann O'Neil / Ann O`Neil & Associates Falls Church / 703-237-9048 www.annoneil.com
Deborah Ogren / Family Centered Resources, Inc. Newport News / 757-596-3941 www.fcr-inc.com
Lundi Palmer / Advocates, Inc. Charlottesville / 434-293-4508
Barbara Payne / ElderCare Strategies, Inc. Ashburn / 703-723-3737 www.eldercarestrategiesinc.com
Sarah Petrick / Aging Gracefully Alexandria / 703-402-0800
Mary Jo Reed / Rehab Inovations Fincastle / 540-473-8699

Maureen Reilly / Assistance for Seniors, Inc. Vienna / 703-319-8787 www.assistanceforseniors.com
Vanessa Rosengart-Bishop / Elder Care Consultants, Inc. Reston / 703-904-0191 www.eldercc.com
Patricia Simpson / Care Connections of VA, LLC Warrenton / 540-347-4181
Stephanie Smith / Senior Advocate, LLC Williamsburg / 757-897-3075 www.senioradvocate.net
Stephanie Thomopoulos / GeriatriCare Management, Inc. Alexandria / 703-313-6114 www.geriatricare.net
Lana Wingate / Care Options for the Elderly & Disabled Williamsburg / 757-259-5949 www.annoneil.com
Emilie Worrall / Independent Aging Resource Center, LLC Charlottesville / 434-296-8916

About the Author

Evan Farr, CELA, CEA, has been in private practice in Fairfax since 1987. As the only attorney in Virginia who is both a Certified Elder Law Attorney and a Certified Estate Advisor, Evan Farr is widely recognized as one of Virginia's leading elder law and estate planning attorneys.

At the local level, Mr. Farr is a member of the Fairfax Bar Association's Elder Law Section and Trusts & Estates Section, and has served in numerous leadership positions within the Association, including Chair of the Election Committee, Chair of the Long Range Planning Committee, and Chair of the Law Practice Management Section.

At the State level, Mr. Farr is a Member of the Board of Directors of National Academy of Elder Law Attorneys Virginia Chapter, and a Council Member of the Virginia Bar Association Elder Law Section.

At the national level, Mr. Farr maintains memberships in the AARP Legal Services Network, the National Academy of Elder Law Attorneys, the National Care Planning Council, and the Gerontological Society of America.

Articles by Mr. Farr in the field of elder law have appeared in numerous publications, including the Guide to Retirement Living (published by Greater Washington Publishing Inc.) and the Golden Gazette (published by the Fairfax County Area Agency on Aging).

Mr. Farr obtained his undergraduate degree in psychology from the University of Pennsylvania in 1984 and received his law degree from the College of William & Mary in 1987.

Mr. Farr's law firm offers a complete range of legal services in connection with elder law and estate planning, including: Medicaid planning, life care planning, long-term care planning, living trusts, wills, powers of attorney, basic and advanced estate planning, private annuities, charitable planning, and business transition planning.

Gaining notoriety as the first Virginia attorney to establish a presence on the World Wide Web when he launched his initial Web site, the Northern Virginia Law Page (www.NorthernVirginiaLawPage.com), during the Summer of 1995, he has since launched two other Virginia legal information Web sites — VirginiaElderLaw.com and VirginiaEstatePlanning.com — both of which have become authoritative resources for Virginia legal consumers.

In his personal life, Mr. Farr is very active in the United Methodist Church and in Scouting. He lives in Clifton with his wife and family.

---

*Virginia has no procedure for approving certifying organizations.